GET THE

NAKED TOOTH

The Truth and Benefits of a

Healthy and Beautiful Smile.

How Dental Implants Can Help You

Live Longer, Smile With Confidence

and Eat the Foods You Want.

by DR. SCOTT HAMBLIN

Publisher:
Elite Online Publishing
63 East 11400 South, #230
Draper, UT 84070
E-mail: info@eliteonlinepublishing.com

ISBN-13: 978-1539387084
ISBN-10: 1539387089

REGISTER

To receive more information, videos and downloads that will help you with Dental Implant Surgery visit:

www.DentalImplantsUtah.com

or

www.TrueDentistry.com

You can also schedule a speaking engagement or consulting session with Dr. Scott Hamblin.

SCOTT HAMBLIN

ABOUT THE AUTHOR

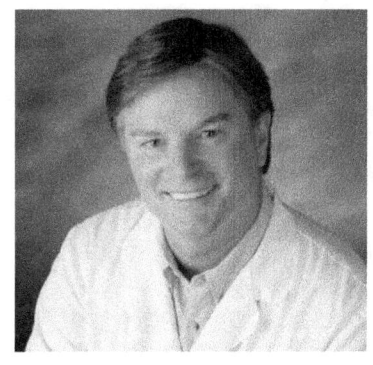

Scott Hamblin, D.D.S. is embracing the dramatic evolutions happening in dental care and treatment, and bringing them to his patients. His goal is to deliver the latest and best practices in ways that are consistent, comfortable and effective for his patients. He has been selected by Consumers Research Council of America as one of America's Top Dentists.

Dr. Hamblin was the team dentist for the Oakland A's professional baseball team for ten years. Dr. Hamblin has over 25 years experience as a practicing dentist in California, Utah, Nevada and Oregon giving him keen insights into what patients are seeking and how leading edge dentistry can fulfill those expectations. As an expert in implants, Dr. Hamblin teaches his techniques nationwide to other dentists. Dr. Hamblin is a graduate of Brigham Young University and Baylor College of Dentistry. His vast experience in aesthetics, implants, and sedation dentistry allows him to use the least invasive techniques and highest quality materials available. Dr. Hamblin is a member of *The International Congress of Oral Implantologists, The American Academy of Implant Dentistry and The American Dental Association.* He is *Invisalign*

Certified and chosen as the *Salt Lake "Extreme Makeover" Dentist*. His unique cosmetic and implant dentistry has been featured on FOX News and ABC.

In his spare time Dr. Hamblin enjoys the outdoors: fly fishing, hiking, tennis, horseback riding, and biking. He also loves traveling with his wife, Linda. He is the father of 6 children and four grandchildren (many more to come!).

CONTENTS

How to Get the Smile You Deserve   1
Oral Health is Directly Related to Overall Health   7
Cosmetic Dentistry   25
Dental Office Team   51
One Doctor, One Office, One Day   77
Comfort Measures   93
Fees and Charges   99
Warranty   107
You Will Look 10 Years Younger!   109
Most Frequently Asked Questions   115

SCOTT HAMBLIN

INTRODUCTION

✓ Do you look in the mirror and see a smile that embarrasses you?

✓ Have you had bad dental experiences in the past?

✓ Do you have MISSING teeth, FAILING teeth or ill-fitting dentures that just don't work?

✓ Are you tired of social embarrassment, not getting noticed by that special someone or looking older than you are?

✓ Do you seriously desire to CHEW COMFORTABLY and knock ten years off your appearance? (Hint: Many of our patients claim that most people rave about how they look like they've "lost weight, gotten a haircut, and look ten years younger" as a bonus from their new smile)

✓ Do you secretly desire to have a bright, white, healthy smile, preserve your existing teeth and live a longer, healthier, happier life?

✓ Are your current dental problems most likely due to putting off dental care because of fear, anxiety, or a busy schedule?

✓ Are you sick and tired of ill-fitting dentures, missing, or worn-out teeth?

If you've answered "YES" to any one of these questions, then this book may just be the most important and emotionally life changing book you've ever read.

What is a Dental Implant?

In a nutshell, a dental implant is a small titanium screw that serves as the replacement for the root portion of a missing natural tooth. A dental implant is an artificial tooth root that is placed into your jaw to hold a replacement tooth or bridge. Dental implants are an option for a person who is missing one or more teeth due to injury, disease or tooth decay. According to statistics, 113 million Americans are missing at least one tooth and 19 million American adults are missing all of their natural teeth.

Dental implants can be placed in either the upper or lower jaws. Where traditional bridges require grinding down healthy tooth structure, dental implants fuse with the bone and become a good anchor for the replacement tooth or teeth. As a result, only individuals with the right amount of natural bone in their jaw are candidates for dental implants.

Baby boomers are turning to Implant Dentistry

Baby boomers revolutionized the disposable diaper industry, and now the baby boomers are doing the same thing for implant dentistry -- revitalizing and recreating it. Baby boomers steadfastly refuse to take aging lying down.

Baby boomers are turning to implant dentistry in droves to restore their youthful smiles. Sturdy dental implants, natural looking veneers, and crowns along with other advances in implant and cosmetic dentistry have much to offer boomers in their quest to turn time back.

Going, going gone are the bridges and messy dentures of yesteryear.

Dental implants are considered more long-lasting and functional than bridges. I have one; my wife has one and I restored my mother's entire upper jaw with dental implants.

Computers are helping dentists perfect their placement of dental implants. Using 3D surgical guides, for example, I can now place dental implants through tiny holes in the gum using a computer to guide me. Then, I can place natural looking porcelain crowns over the implant.

What about crowns?

Today's crowns are much better than crowns of the past. The all new ceramic crowns, which are metal free, do not show that tell-tale gray line at the base of the gums, so no-one can tell they are not your natural choppers.

How about that smile?

SCOTT HAMBLIN

A smile is more than skin deep

No matter how old (or young you are), part of a doing a proper smile makeover is making sure the dentist is knowledgeable in cosmetic and implant dentistry. You want to be able to eat with, brush and floss these teeth and live with them for years to come. I have 25 years or more of experience and I love to make smiles beautiful.

1

HOW TO GET THE SMILE YOU DESERVE

The Smile that Lights Up a Room

Everyone you talk to agrees that a great smile is truly one of the best assets in life. You've even heard people say it, "She has got such beautiful teeth. When she smiles, it lights up the room."

Now, wouldn't you like that said about your smile?

Proven by science, a great smile is not purely vanity or being selfish.

It is about getting the absolute most out of life and helping all those around you do the same. Before we get too far down the road, let's talk about the one true negative; it costs money to get a great smile. Honestly, whether you consider this a cost or investment in yourself depends on what you consider important in life.

For some people, it will simply never be worth much to them- it is truly a cost.

For most folks, once they look at what's really important, they feel that the expense of a great smile is an investment in their well-being. Like clockwork, an investment in your smile will pay huge dividends 24 hours a day/7 days a week.

"I was always comfortable during my procedures. Right now, I am more pleased with my smile and my overall dental health than I ever thought possible. What I love about the continuing care at Dr. Hamblin's is how professional everyone is and how friendly. If I knew of someone to be helped I'd urge them to see Dr. Hamblin--- I'm glad I did!"
Jessica, Waitress, Sandy, Utah

A great smile makes a difference in your life every minute of every hour. For some people, it even makes a difference while they sleep. (If you are wearing dentures or are missing any teeth you may be one of those people that will benefit from dental implants 24 hours a day.)

The question is, how worth it is it to you? Every individual must decide just how valuable and important a great smile is to him or herself.

I will give you a hint: What if your pay went up 12.5-14.25 percent? Here's a quick exercise to tell you how much a smile may be worth to you. Go ahead and multiply your salary by the additional percentage of pay; be conservative and use the 12.5%. Now multiply that additional amount of pay times the number of years you plan to continue working. For someone that makes $30,000 a year that intends to retire in 20 years, the additional pay just for having a beautiful smile for those 20 years could be worth at least $75,000 in today's dollars.

Other enormous benefits such as increased self-confidence, greater self-esteem, enhanced personal and business relationships and being treated better by those around you, make more friends and business contacts easier. Having an increased ability to influence your associates, colleagues, customers, friends and even the next door neighbor tips the scale overwhelmingly (bang!) to the side of having a great smile. Now don't you agree that this investment pays dividends every day of your life? For many people it is not an option, it is truly a necessity.

People Always Look At Your Teeth. What do they see?

It is scientifically proven that the first or second thing people notice when they look at you is your smile or teeth. Did you realize this? Some studies show it is the eyes first and the smile second while others the results are vice versa. Either way, when you come into contact with other people, they ARE going to notice your teeth and smile no matter what. The main ways people communicate with other people are with their mouths and eyes.

People are drawn to beautiful things and having a beautiful smile is hugely important in how attractive you are to other people. You probably already knew this by having common sense but over the past 20-30 years, the scientific evidence has gradually proven the importance of a great smile and how you are perceived and treated by others in every situation in life.

Attractiveness Determines How Other People Perceive and Treat You in All Situations

What has science proven? The bottom line is this: the better you look, the better you are treated by others. It cannot be emphasized enough that being more attractive has distinct advantages. Generally, people greatly underestimate this reality. Like it or not, people who are seen by others as attractive are thought to be smarter, better at their jobs, more talented, more kind, and even more honest!

This concept is true throughout our entire society at every level. Your smile and teeth play a large part in how many other people want to be around you and how much they like and believe you. Just by having a great smile you become more likely to be promoted in your job, more attractive and likely to find your best mate in life, more likely to be wanted by others in friendships, and even more likely to be trusted.

What are the Social Advantages of Looking Good?

People that are good-looking enjoy huge social advantages without even trying. They are seen as smarter and liked better. They are seen as more desirable and to have better personalities. Nice looking people have an ability to persuade those around them and are far more likely to receive help from others.

Attractive School Children Get Into Less Trouble in School and Are Seen As Being Smarter

A study by Dion in 1972 showed that attractive school children were viewed as less naughty when misbehaving compared to children that were less attractive. In 1992, a study by Ritts, Patterson, and Tabbs, found that teachers perceive attractive students as more intelligent than less attractive students.

Good-Looking Political Candidates Are More Likely to Win Elections

Few people would admit to voting for a candidate because he/she were more attractive. A Canadian study proved this bias (Efran and Patterson in 1976). Political candidates that were attractive got two and a half more times the number of votes compared to unattractive candidates. Voters, of course, denied that their votes were influenced by whether a candidate was good looking or not, yet it is true.

Attractiveness Influences the Law and Justice System: Being Attractive Means Less Severe Penalties

A study in Pennsylvania in 1980 by Steward showed good-looking people received more favorable treatment in the justice system, and that attractive people were far more likely to avoid jail time, and if they did receive a jail sentence, it was much lighter.

Being Attractive Makes Getting Jobs Easier

A 1990 study (Mack and Rainey) showed that being nice looking and well-groomed accounted more in the hiring decision than job qualifications!

You Can Make More Money If You Have a Great Smile

Attractive workers get paid on average up to 14% more than unattractive workers. This was shown to be true in both the U.S. and Canada.

"I am so glad Dr. Hamblin fixed my teeth. I have received 2 job promotions in just 2 weeks immediately after having my teeth fixed. Before, I would never smile, because I was embarrassed and I am sure my customers and managers thought I was upset all the time. Now, I just smile all the time! Having a beautiful, sexy smile has opened many doors for me.

-Susan, Cosmetics Sales Rep, Salt Lake City, Utah

Men and Women Agree That Attractive Teeth Are Better

Both sexes respond to attractiveness in the same ways. Having a better smile makes you better in all kinds of ways to both men and women.

2

ORAL HEALTH IS DIRECTLY RELATED TO OVERALL HEALTH

Did you know that your oral health can offer clues about your overall health and the problems in your mouth can affect the rest of your body? What is the connection between oral health and overall health? Like many areas of the body your mouth is teeming with bacteria, most of them harmless. Typically the body's natural defenses and good oral health care such as daily brushing and flossing can keep these bacteria under control. Bacteria can reach high levels that lead to oral infections such as tooth decay and gum disease without proper oral health.

Quality of life = health, wealth, and teeth!

Having life's cake and being able to eat it comfortably, is a goal we all share. How much does losing teeth change the quality of life?

Since the primary function of teeth is chewing, tooth loss can reduce chewing ability that leads to detrimental changes in food selection. This, in turn, may increase the risk of particular diseases since diet and individual health states, such as cardiovascular health, are linked. For example, an increase in cholesterol and saturated fat, and a decrease in fiber have been shown to elevate the risk of heart disease. Since a **large portion of the population has missing teeth,** the effect on health risks due to tooth loss may have a significant impact.

In what is one of the largest studies investigating a relationship between tooth loss and diet, data was collected on the dental status and food and nutrient intake from over 49,000 male professionals. The findings indicate that intake of vegetables, fiber and carotene was significantly lower, while intake of total calories, cholesterol and fat were significantly higher in participants with no teeth compared to participants with 25 teeth or more.

In a follow-up study with the same group, a comparison between tooth loss and consumption of specific foods and nutrients were performed. The findings show over an eight-year period, participants without any tooth loss had reductions in daily intake of saturated fat, cholesterol, and vitamin B12, and increases in daily intake of fiber, carotene and fruits compared to participants with tooth loss.Also, subjects who lost five or more teeth were significantly more likely to stop eating apples, pears, and carrots compared to subjects who lost four teeth or less.

These studies provide the best evidence to date for an association between tooth loss and a change in food intake and the health risks of a poor diet.

Researchers reported in a study published in a recent issue of American Journal of Preventive Medicine that there is a high, progressive association between tooth loss and heart disease. The table below documents the results.

Amount of Tooth Loss	Percentage of Heart Disease
No tooth loss	4.7%
Missing 1-5 Teeth	5.7%
Missing 6-31 Teeth	8.5%

The results are consistent with previous studies that link gum disease and tooth loss to an increased risk of atherosclerosis and heart disease.

More than 120 medical conditions, some of them life-threatening, can be detected in the early stages by a dentist. A high percentage of health conditions are documented to have oral symptoms, such as swollen or bleeding gums, ulcers, dry mouth, bad breath, metallic taste and various other changes in the oral cavity.

A report from Scientific American indicates a relationship between oral and overall physical health with many organs or systems in the body being affected. The connection between some specific health conditions and oral health should be the reason you promote good oral health for you and your family.

Periodontal "Gum" Disease

Periodontal disease is a chronic inflammatory disease caused by more than 500 bacterial species found in plaque below the gum line. Periodontal disease a fancy term for gum disease including gingivitis can cause swollen gums, irritation, and bleeding. A more advanced form called periodontitis can lead to receding gums, damaged tissue and bone around the teeth and even tooth loss. Periodontal disease is the sixth most prevalent chronic condition in the world affecting seven hundred and forty-three million people in the United States alone it affects one in every two adults and two and a half times more people than diabetes.

Gum disease affects nearly 50 percent of Americans, many of whom don't know they have it, because, in the early stages, it is painless. One study found that people with higher blood levels of bacteria in the mouth were more likely to have a build-up of plaque in the carotid artery in the neck (a blockage there can lead to stroke).

Periodontal disease is now recognized by the Cardiology community to be a direct risk factor for coronary artery disease, peripheral artery disease, and stroke. Last November, the American Society of Kidney Specialist or Nephrology presented a study showing that African-Americans with normal kidney functions but with severe periodontal disease went on to develop chronic kidney disease at four times the rate as those without severe periodontal disease.

In 2012, the American Heart Association released a statement acknowledging the association between gum disease and cardiovascular disease. The Cardiology community recognizes periodontal disease as a risk factor for coronary artery disease, peripheral artery disease, and stroke.

Inflammation is the leading suspect--it underlies gum disease as well as heart disease, diabetes, arthritis, cancer, Alzheimer's disease and more. Bottom line: if you have periodontal disease, you could be vulnerable to a long list of scary medical problems that could cut your life short.

Gingivitis is a gum disease that can cause all kinds of issues in our months including destroying the gum and bone that support and anchor teeth. Gingivitis is the major contributor to the loss of teeth and leads to periodontal disease. A periodontal disease is where calculus, better known as tartar, builds up on the gum line and under the gums. Moreover, must be removed from under the gum line. If not the infection eats away at the jaw bone.

What are the warning signs of gum disease?

A dental examination is usually when people learn they have gum disease. Heart disease can creep up on you silently and so can gum disease. Gum disease is sneaky and symptoms may not show up until it is too late. The early warning signs can be silent. Here are the warning signs:

- Red, swollen or tender gums or other mouth pain.

- Your gums bleed when you brush, floss or eat hard food

- Your gums are pulling away from your teeth (your teeth look longer than they used to)

- Loose or separating teeth

- Pus between your gums and teeth

- Sores in your mouth

- Persistent bad breath

- A change in your bite (the way your teeth fit together)

- Foul taste in your mouth

After a patient experiences pain and visible symptoms, many times the disease has progressed to its advanced stages.

"Gum disease is as bad for your heart as high blood pressure and high cholesterol. Because it has few warning signs, most people do not know they have gum disease until their dentist tells them," says Robert Pick, a spokesman for the American Dental Association.

Bacteria in Your Mouth are Linked To Diseases

Bacteria which cause serious dental problems, such as *gum disease*, have been identified as potential causative factors for health conditions such as diabetes, high blood pressure, and even coronary artery disease. In fact, some studies have shown that men over 50 who have gum disease have a 72% increased risk for coronary artery disease (CAD). You read that right, 72%!

Research has shown that chronic gum disease and bleeding gums can introduce over *700* different kinds of bacteria into the bloodstream. At least some of those bacteria are known to produce an enzyme which causes inflammation in the arteries, which results in CAD. High blood pressure and other inflammatory diseases have been linked to pathologic oral bacteria entering the bloodstream.

Diseases Caused By Gum Disease

Periodontal (Gum) Disease affects 75% of American Adults. It is the leading cause of adult tooth loss and cost Americans millions of dollars in dental care every year. The recent developments which point to gum disease and destructive oral bacteria as a cause of severe health conditions make it even more important to practice good dental hygiene, see your dentist twice per year, and take action to prevent and reverse the progression of gum disease. Make certain gum disease do not destroy more than just your smile. Gum Disease can cause Oral Cancer, Cavities, Inflammation, Heart Disease, Diabetes, Osteoporosis, Low Birth Weight and Poor Oral Health in Children.

Oral Cancer

Oral cancers are a real threat to our mouths. Regular exams by your dentist can be a life-saving health benefit. Signs of oral cancers include sores that do not heal, unusual bleeding or white patches on gums. Regular tissue and gum examinations will ensure that your oral tissues are healthy and that you have no malignant tissues that may require biopsies.

Cavities

Cavities are not only painful but can become a serious health threat when left untreated. Cavities can cause infections, which, in turn, can cause problems for the other supporting structures in our mouths. Infections in the mouth can also potentially spread to the bloodstream, leading to a condition known as septicemia. Septicemia is a serious life threatening infection that can get worse very quickly. It can arise from infections in the mouth and throughout the body. Early detection of cavities can save pain, money and prevent health problems.

Inflammation

Experts have said that inflammation makes us more susceptible to aging and disease.Also persistent, systemic inflammation appears to be at the root of all known chronic health conditions. You can help yourself live a longer healthier life by doing your part to prevent any inflammation in your body. Since inflammation is a threat in the mouth, proper care and dental check-ups are key to living long and healthy lives. Your dentist is an excellent source of information and prevention of any problematic inflammation in your mouth. Regular checkups are the way you preserve your good oral and overall health and help you live longer and better!

Cardiovascular and Heart Disease

Diseases are linked to poor oral health. For example, Endocarditis, an in-fection of the inner lining of your heart. Bacteria or other germs from other parts of your body such as your mouth spread to the bloodstream and attach to damaged areas in your heart. Poor oral health is linked to car-diovascular disease. Some research suggests that heart disease, clogged ar-teries, and stroke might be related to the inflammation and infections that oral bacteria can cause.

The same bacteria that cause periodontal disease also trigger an immune response, inflammation, which causes the arteries to swell. The swelling of the arterial walls results in a constriction of blood flow that can lead to a higher incidence of cardiovascular disease.

Dr. Weston Price, DDS, presented similar information in the early 1930s. His discoveries made comparable observations that bacteria found in the oral cavity did indeed circulate throughout the entire body. Not only could it lead to a higher incidence of cardiovascular disease but it also causes a degenerative condition to exist for all your major organ systems.

If people, especially women, could reduce their risk of stroke, heart attacks and heart problems by a third then that would be a breakthrough. Heart attacks and strokes kill more women than breast cancer, so decreasing that risk by 33 percent is something you should pursue. Get an appointment with your dentist and have him evaluate your mouth for gum disease.

The exact mechanism of how gum disease may be linked to heart disease and stroke is unclear. One thought is that poor dental hygiene leads to an overgrowth of oral bacteria. These organisms, fairly benign in the mouth, can get into the bloodstream through the gums and, once there, they can clump on blood vessel walls and grow into plaques that clog arteries and lead to heart attacks and strokes. Moreover, because these bacteria are foreign to the body, once they infiltrate the bloodstream, blood vessels think they are being attacked and try to kill them, just as they would an infection. This results in inflammation and swelling that narrows blood vessels and prevents adequate blood flow to vital organs like the brain and heart.

The recent study was less concerned with the details of why gum disease increases the risk of heart disease and stroke, but whether the risk can be reduced through frequent dental visits.

"Poor oral hygiene has been associated with increased risk of cardiovascular disease," the study's abstract acknowledged. "However, the association between preventive dentistry and cardiovascular risk reduction remained underdetermined."

Dr. Zu-Yin Chen and colleagues at Taipei Veterans General Hospital in Taiwan followed more than 100,000 patients over a seven-year period, only half of whom had ever had their teeth cleaned. They found that the participants who had their teeth cleaned, even only once, lowered the risk of a heart attack and a 13 percent lower stroke risk compared to those who had never had a dental cleaning.

Not only did dental cleanings reduce the risk of heart disease and stroke, but Chen said in the news release, "Protection from heart disease and stroke was more pronounced in participants who got tooth scaling at least once a year." The press release said that people that had their teeth cleaned, the lower their risk of heart disease and stroke.

Although the results suggest that preventative dental care can lower risk of heart disease and stroke, the study did not account for other cardiovascular risk factors that could have contributed to the association.

"We cannot lose sight of the fact that most heart attacks and strokes are related to the so-called traditional risk factors, and those are high blood pressure, high cholesterol, high blood sugar, smoking, weighing too much and not exercising enough. It remains very important to take control of those risk factors," said Gerber. "People shouldn't think that by going to the dentist more often they're going to reduce their risk of heart disease."

Periodontal disease results in higher levels of body inflammation that can be measured with blood tests of the inflammatory proteins and cells. These blood tests are CRP, TNF-a, IL-6, the white blood count, and sedimentation rate (2). These inflammatory markers when chronically elevated are also associated with atrial fibrillation and abnormal heart rhythm in the upper heart chambers, coronary atherosclerosis, and risk of myocardial infarction or a heart attack (3, 4). In fact, the bacteria found in the mouth that causes periodontal disease have also been found in the atherosclerotic plaques of people with coronary artery disease (5). This last finding suggests that heart harm can be caused not only by the body's reaction to the disease in the mouth but from the bacterium invading the body itself.

At the annual meeting of the American Society for Microbiology in May, researchers from the University of Florida and University of British Columbia presented further evidence of a connection. A six-month experiment involving mice infected with four different types of bacteria known to cause gum disease, showed the mice having an increased inflammation and cholesterol levels which are both linked to cardiovascular disease. In addition, the bacteria traveled to the mice hearts, kidneys, lungs, and livers.

Diabetes

Poor oral health has been associated with diabetes. Diabetes reduces the body's resistance to infection putting the gums at risk. Gum disease appears to be more frequent and severe among people who have diabetes. Research shows that individuals who have gum disease have a harder time controlling their blood sugar levels.

Besides the risk of developing CAD or other cardiovascular disease, gum disease has been linked to diabetes. In fact, evidence strongly suggests that patients who have both diabetes and gum disease can more easily control one disease when the other disease is under control. That means that keeping your blood sugar in check will help manage gum disease, and improving the health of your gums will help you control your blood sugar.

Osteoporosis

Osteoporosis, which causes bones to become weak and brittle, might be linked with periodontal bone loss and tooth loss. Tooth loss before the age of 35 might be a risk factor for Alzheimer's disease as well.

Poor Oral Health in Children

Oral health, in general, is declining. Children with severe oral diseases may have difficulty chewing and may not eat enough or may have modified diets that do not contain the nutrients required for healthy growth and development.

Children with severe oral disease may be reluctant to smile due to embarrassment about the appearance of their teeth. The lack of a smile can cause low self-esteem. Some infants and children with severe oral disease may have difficulty sleeping and infants and children with severe oral disease may have frequent absences from school. Currently, tooth decay is the number one reason why children miss school.

Premature or Low Birth Weight

Poor oral health has been determined to cause premature birth and low birth weight.

Treatment of Gum Disease

The gums should not bleed if you brush or floss regularly. A sign of gum disease is bleeding, infection and inflammation. Getting your teeth cleaned regularly and flossing your teeth often will make the gums healthier. The more you mechanically stimulate the gums, the more bacteria that will get killed and the inflammation will go away. Gum disease is not treatable, but is stoppable, but once the bone loss has occurred, there is little opportunity to grow new bone. The only treatment is stopping the gum disease from getting worse. Gum disease leads to tooth loss, dentures and then dental implants.

One of the biggest advancements in dentistry has been the dental laser. It is a laser that we use to treat gum disease. In the past, the dental team would clean everything out of the mouth mechanically or physically by removing the tartar and the bacteria off the teeth. Currently, patients with gum disease have their teeth scaled and cleaned, and the pockets disinfected with the laser at the spot where the gum disease is. The technique works wonders as far as treating gum disease.

In addition to dental implants, diode lasers, and treating teeth with ozone are significant advancements in the last twenty years. The tooth is flooded with ozone which kills all the bacteria and stops the decay process. The deeper, bigger cavities still have to be cleaned out to remove the decay, but if treated with ozone it guarantees that there are no bacteria left in the tooth. The filling or crown will have a clean surface.

Healthy Habits

Being more diligent about brushing, flossing and seeing the dentist, can save your life since research shows that if gum disease is treated, blood vessel health can improve in as little as six months.

Researchers now suggest that by having our teeth professionally cleaned and scraped even just once, we can help reduce our risk of heart attack and stroke. Chronic inflammation is behind this association. Regular cleaning and scaling reduces inflammation-causing bacteria and improves blood vessel function. Experts have linked inflammation in our bodies to contributing to many diseases, especially cardiovascular disease.

Here are some tips that may take you to the next level of oral care:

- Brush your teeth twice a day, in the morning and before you go to bed.

- Use fluoride toothpaste

- Make sure you brush the back as well as the front of your teeth.

- Brush your tongue. The whitish coating you see in the morning is plaque that can cause bad breath and is a breeding ground for bacteria.

- Get an electric toothbrush. The back and forth action of the brush head works better to remove plaque than a manual toothbrush. Most are timed to signal when you've brushed for two minutes; three is better.

- Use an antiseptic mouthwash, or a fluoride or anti-plaque mouthwash.

- Floss at least once a day; get between all your teeth and move the floss up and down several times

- Buy some disclosing tablets at the drugstore--you chew them, and they highlight any plaque that you missed in brushing.

- See your dentist regularly for checkups and professional teeth cleaning.

- Eat foods that protect against plaque and harmful sugars: cheeses, peanuts, yogurt, and milk.

- Avoid sticky sweet foods--prolonged contact can damage teeth. Avoid bedtime snacks unless you want to brush your teeth again.

A habit that takes five minutes a day can add years to your life. It also helps prevent everything from heart attacks and strokes to diabetes, colds, flu, and arthritis. What's more, it even improves your looks and fights bad breath.

A new study published in *Journal of Aging Research* adds to mounting evidence that one of the simplest, and cheapest, secrets of long life is taking care of your teeth, with daily brushing and flossing. Conversely, neglecting your teeth, skipping dental visits, can be fatal.

To protect your oral health, practice good oral hygiene every day. Brush your teeth at least twice a day, floss daily, eat a healthy diet and limit in-between meals snacks. Replace your toothbrush every three or four months or sooner if bristles are frayed and schedule regular dental checkups.

At a recent dental education course, Dr. Dunn and his Dental Hygienist, Melody studied the pathologic effects of these bacteria and how to identify them through *saliva testing*. Many dentists treat oral bacteria and the inflammatory processes of gum disease only after symptoms like reddening, swollen or bleeding gums manifest. Prevention is now more important than ever. Currently, you can have painless testing performed right in the dental office to detect destructive bacteria. The bacteria can damage your teeth and gums as well as damage your heart. Detecting and treating this infection can help you stay healthier longer.

A study from the University of California, Berkeley, found that women who see a dentist twice a year cut their risk of stroke, heart attacks, and other cardiovascular problems by at least a third. It is no secret that taking care of your pearly whites is good for your heart. Bacteria from gum disease may enter your bloodstream and trigger an immune response that causes arteries to swell, constrict, and collect plaque, all of which increase your chance of having heart problems. Your healthy habits at home are not the only thing that counts.

Going to the dentist twice a year is what the study correlated to the benefits. By simply showing up and having your teeth cleaned and your oral habits evaluated seems to make the difference.

If you have the beginning of gum disease, start with a plan to manage the treatment and change the habits that make it worse. In the meantime, floss daily and brush effectively. Typical mouthwashes kill 99.9 percent of oral bacteria, but only for about 20 minutes. Your dentist can prescribe an inexpensive mouthwash that kills the same 99.9 percent of dangerous bacteria, but for eight hours.

If you smoke and value your gums and teeth, don't smoke. Using tobacco multiplies your risk of gum disease by six makes it harder to treat and raises the risk of tooth loss.

Good-bye, "morning breath" and "hello!" to a healthier mouth and HEART, no matter what your age!

Americans are *NOT* regular flossers. It is estimated that only 5% to 10% of Americans regularly floss. According to studies done at Emory University by the Centers for Disease Control and Prevention, common gum problems such as gingivitis and periodontitis lead to a 23% – 46% higher rate of death.

If that does not get your attention, are you aware that daily flossing adds an average of 6.3 years to a person's lifespan? That is right! According to Michael F. Roizen, MD in his book, Real Age, he writes that "flossing your teeth daily can make your arteries younger. Studies show that flossing helps keep your immune system young."

In the 1940s, a German scientist named, Reinhardt Voll, MD also made a very profound statement, "80 – 90% of all ailments in the body originate in the oral cavity." If you can eliminate the presence of unwanted bacteria in the mouth by simply flossing before you brush your teeth, then you are providing yourself an excellent opportunity to stay healthy and even live longer.

For all of you "non-flossers", I want to make a personal challenge to each and every one of you. Find a pack of floss, or buy some floss or even send me an e-mail and I'll send you some floss for free. Carefully floss around all your teeth (takes 2 minutes or less) making sure that you are getting the floss below the gum line and then visually examine your gums in the mirror after you are finished.

Most likely you'll see your gums bleeding or feel the blood in your mouth. If so, read the following information very carefully. If your gums are bleeding:

- There is an inflammatory response taking place in your mouth with harmful bacteria entering the bloodstream.

- Your immune system is stressed.

- The health of the primary organ systems is compromised, such as the heart, kidneys, lungs, stomach, liver, gallbladder, adrenals, spleen, large and small intestines. Everything gets exposed from this bacteria originating in the mouth.

In a trial of approximately 300 patients seen in cardiac or heart clinics, and referred for community dental care, were randomized to aggressive dental care and hygiene versus the patient's standard dental care. Those that received aggressive care for their periodontal disease had lower levels of body inflammation at six months, and this was felt to be associated with a lower risk of heart disease progression (6). Unfortunately, to date, no studies have shown that aggressive periodontal care can reduce the risk of worsening of cardiovascular disease. Right now this is assumed since body inflammation results in worsening cardiovascular disease and treatment of periodontal disease reduce body inflammation.

Impact on Life and Longevity

California researchers tracked 5,611 seniors for 17 years, and found that:

- Not brushing at night boosted the risk of death during the study period by 20 to 35 percent, compared to brushing every night.

- Never flossing increased mortality risk by 30 percent, versus daily flossing.

- Not seeing a dentist in the previous 12 months raised the risk of death by up to 50 percent, compared to getting dental care two or more times a year.

Another startling finding: One major predictor of early death was missing teeth, even after other risk factors were taken into account, the study reported. People who wore dentures had a 30 percent higher mortality risk than those with 20 or more remaining teeth.

3

COSMETIC DENTISTRY

Will you look better in addition to chewing better?

Cosmetic dentistry has the ability to enhance a person's smile while still retaining the natural look of a smile, so nobody knows the person enhanced their teeth. Cosmetic dentistry may include the following:

- Bonding, Porcelain veneers, crowns, dental implants

- Laser gum surgery

- Teeth whitening, laser whitening

- Orthodontics, Invisalign™

Utilizing cosmetic dentistry on a patient should provide the "wow" factor. When people look at your patient, they should think or say "wow that smile looks great!" It looks white; it looks healthy, but it looks natural. Even if the patient has fake teeth, the teeth should not be too white like toilet bowl porcelain. The teeth should look natural, not fake or out of place.

Cosmetic dentistry is kind of all over the spectrum. The treatment can range from twenty- somethings with big gaps in between their teeth to dentures and dental implants. The point is the patient is not confident when they smile. The patient may have experienced a cosmetic dentistry that was less than perfect. The patient may just want a perfect smile for portraits.

Cosmetic Dentistry allows the patient to smile with confidence and chew or eat whatever they want. Also, the patient should look natural, better, healthier, and younger. After the procedure, there should be the "wow" effect so that the patient has friends and family telling them they look at least ten years younger. The work should never look fake, only natural.

One patient in particular who was a cosmetic representative in a major department store had broken snaggly teeth and never improved the teeth. She noticed it was affecting her career. Other employees were getting advancements and perks. She wanted her smile restored to look prettier and healthier. Her smile consisted of teeth that were chipped, broken or decayed. We put temporaries for a couple of weeks while we waited for the final porcelain crowns to be done. In the two week period, she got a promotion because she was smiling all the time and attracted more customers. She was ecstatic and jubilant. After we had put her final porcelain teeth, she got another promotion within a month. The quality of life improved while her beautiful looking smile helped her career.

Some people have genetically bad teeth or soft teeth if you will. My mom has bad teeth, and my dad has great teeth. I, unfortunately, inherited my mom's teeth, so I have had root canals, dental implants, crowns, and fillings. I've had it all, and I brush and floss my teeth like three or four times a day. My friend who is a dentist in California never flosses his teeth, and he has never had a cavity at all

The decay in your front teeth and may be caused if the teeth are not aligned properly. I had one patient who had lots of tooth decay. I do not know what caused the rapid decay. Some dentists call it "meth mouth" or "Mountain Dew mouth" named after sugared soda. Cola or Mountain Dew seem to soften the teeth and weaken the teeth and cause more tooth decay. Just drink water and not much will go wrong with your teeth as a result.

I have had some patients come in with rotten teeth. It is so rewarding to fix those patient's teeth and give them a beautiful smile. They smile broadly and confidently and you know they might get job promotions or meet their soul mate. The point is they have confidence they did not have before.

Porcelain Veneers

Porcelain veneers are made up of medical-grade ceramic that is attached to the front surfaces of teeth for smile transformation. The veneers are custom made for each patient and closely resembled the appearance of natural tooth enamel.

One of my patients was a waitress working at Texas Roadhouse. She had significant gaps in her teeth but was a very attractive girl. When she smiled is when you noticed her teeth. She always had the gaps. We put porcelain veneers on her and closed up all those spaces. Her smile is beautiful and inside you know she feels great.

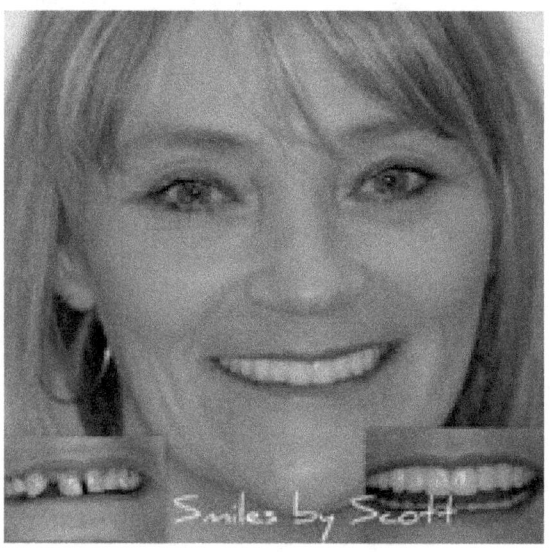

I've done porcelain veneers on my adult children. Five of my six children have porcelain veneers on their front teeth as well as my wife. The family portraits show the entire family with great smiles, and I am so proud I was able to make their smiles beautiful.

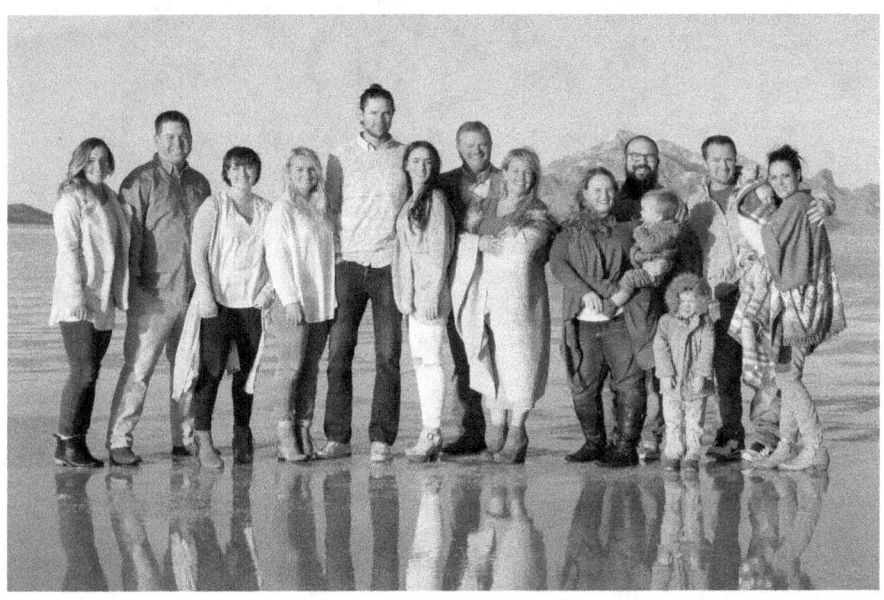

I did my wife's porcelain veneers over ten years ago. For most of my cosmetic cases, I utilized a local laboratory here in Utah. The laboratory does fantastic work, and all the cosmetic cases I did were amazing. The porcelain veneers look natural; they look good, but I wanted to find the best laboratory in the country. So, I called a few professional friends and found a lab in Beverly Hills, California. The lab is very expensive, but supposedly did the best work; I sent my wife's case there.

The first time the porcelain veneers looked unnatural, so I sent the

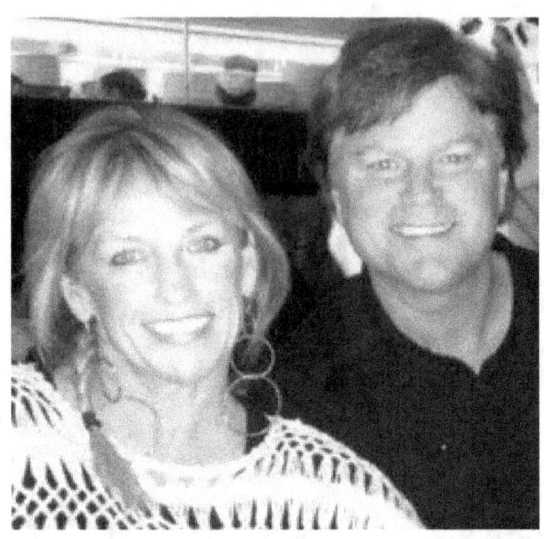

impression back, and they did the work again. The second time, the work was better, so I went ahead and bonded the porcelain veneers to her teeth. Every time I looked at them, the porcelain veneers did not look natural. The teeth were not translucent enough, and my wife agreed. I ended up taking them all back off and sending them to the local laboratory here in Utah. The first time they came back, they were perfect. Her smile is fantastic, and I love it.

New "Age-Erasing Dentures"

Sometimes you get dentures, and they do not fit right, or they are not for your facial structures, and they look 'fake'.. Until now, you have had the choice of the inexpensive set that had plastic teeth and did not fit very well or an expensive custom denture which usually fit better. But, you still looked like you were wearing a denture.

Finally, some tools and techniques were developed for age-erasing or facelift like features, which can now be applied to dentures. I offer a third option, a new kind of denture called *Age-Erasing Dentures*.

The basis for this new type of denture is called neuromuscular treatment. Because your dentures rest partially on the muscles in your jaw, neuromuscular dentistry makes sure to find the position of your optimum muscle relaxation and function. If we can achieve stable and relaxed muscles before we take impressions for your dentures, you will automatically get a better fit.

Most patients do not realize that once their teeth are removed, jawbone deterioration begins. Because the typical behaviors of biting and chewing cause the root of the tooth to physically stimulate the bone, once that root is removed the stimulation stops, and the bone begins to deteriorate.

As long as natural teeth are in place and disease is absent, your upper and lower jaws can be expected to remain healthy and intact. However the loss of your teeth and the placement of traditional dentures, which are designed to rest on top of the gum tissue, do not provide direct stimulation to the jaw bone and thus do nothing to combat the effects of jawbone resorption. The patient looks much older than they are.

My *Age-Erasing Dentures* are designed to stimulate the jawbone by creating a better fitting denture that rests partially on the muscles. They are placed to build your "**bite**" at a position which best supports your muscle function. The position also provides stronger facial support, which in turn, creates a more youthful look.

Of course, this is the most expensive type of denture, but this denture will be comfortable, it will fit, and it will give you a beautiful smile. I still recommend implants over these types of dentures.

I recognized that my patients who needed dentures were not happy with teeth that looked artificial. I have perfected a system that makes sure the dentures placed were beautiful and natural-looking as well as comfortable and functional.

These *Age-Erasing Dentures* appear more natural because they are designed and handcrafted especially to complement your personality, age, sex, and physical appearance. When you elect to have these, *Age-Erasing Dentures* we take extraordinary measures to make sure that your smile is incredible."

When you come to me for dentures, I partner with you at every step of the way to ensure you receive the exact smile makeover you want. I cannot wait for you to see your new smile and work very hard to make sure everything is perfect.

I offer more than just an attractive denture that will enhance your appearance. These dentures are also designed to provide better chewing and biting than normal dentures. Although nothing compares to healthy natural teeth, a secured set of implanted teeth come in second place.

All of our Age-Erasing Dentures:

- Feature teeth that are individually handset to give you that youthful, natural look

- Match in tooth size to the size of your face

- Give you choices in tooth shape and color

- Make sure that your new smile is naturally your own. I compared photographs of you before you lost your teeth to make sure that your new smile is naturally your own.

Our denture patients enjoy the ability to flash an incredible smile while wearing a denture that provides stability, optimal chewing efficiency, and comfort.

I make sure the dentures you receive are exquisite and matched perfectly to your face. Quite simply, my goal is to create dentures for you that make you look and feel like your ultimate self.

Teeth play a vital role in defining who you are. They give each face a unique identity, just as the eyes and nose make each face distinctive and easily recognized. Your natural teeth were unique in size, shape, arrangement, and in the support, they gave your lips and cheeks.

The closer we can get the artificial teeth to how your natural teeth were, the more you look and feel like your old self. Our goal in setting your artificial teeth, is to place them where the natural teeth were. When we do this, your bite looks and feels natural. You can smile without feeling self-conscious, and you can eat the foods that you like comfortably and normally.

I use custom dentures to craft your *Age-Erasing Dentures*. With the custom fit and design, with your new dentures, you will get both a beautifully natural smile and improved chewing function. (But nothing compared to healthy natural teeth, or implanted solid teeth.)

My dentures will give you a gorgeous, natural-looking smile.

If you look closely at someone with a beautiful smile and straight teeth, you will notice that each tooth is not precisely aligned with its neighbor tooth. Instead, the placement of the teeth varies slightly to create a beautiful and natural smile line.

I am a *Cosmetic Artist*. I have practiced my craft for over 25 years. I will use every tool and possible resource to make sure that your dentures are not just "fine." I will make sure your dentures are nothing short of amazing. As part of that procedure, you can expect the following:

- Match the tooth size to the size of your face. All too often, artificial teeth can look exactly like "artificial." Off the shelf teeth could be too large for your face, or too small. Either way, they call attention to themselves and don't look right. I will make sure that your new teeth fit your face, perfectly.

- I give you choices in tooth shape and color. No one knows your mouth and your teeth like you do. For each tooth, you will choose from a variety of shapes, sizes, and colors. Whether you want to replicate your old smile or enhance it in your new one, I will help you choose teeth that will be uniquely right for you.

- I spend time with you and get to know you. Your distinct personality should be reflected in your smile. You'll want to look and feel like yourself when you smile, and that is exactly what I want, too.

- I ask for photos of you before you lost your teeth. It is important to me that when you smile, you look like you. By looking at your pictures, I can be sure to match size, shape and placement of your new teeth.

- I hand set each tooth. For most dentures, the teeth are placed in the lab, not by a dentist who can look at you in his office, and who knows your teeth and your smile well. I will handset each of your new teeth, making sure to get each one as closely as possible to where your natural teeth were. Your new teeth will look and feel natural.

- If possible, I utilize pre-extraction dental records to aid in tooth placement.

- I make sure that your dentures are secure. Me and my team are experienced in the most advanced techniques available to secure your dentures and keep them comfortable.

- If you qualify, I can secure your dentures using *dental implants* or *mini-implants*. I perform these surgical procedures in the comfort of my office.

These dental restorations are a hybrid of complete dentures and dental implants. Dentures sit on top of implanted posts using four or more dental implants as an anchor. Dental restoration security is achieved allowing the dentures to move naturally with the jawbone.

You can chew through tougher foods and smile with confidence, knowing your dentures will not slip.

Virtual Face Lift from Implant Supported Dentures. Here is a before and after picture of a patient showing the age-reducing effects:

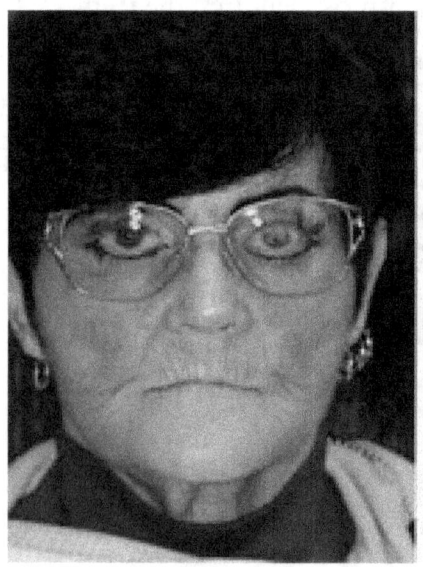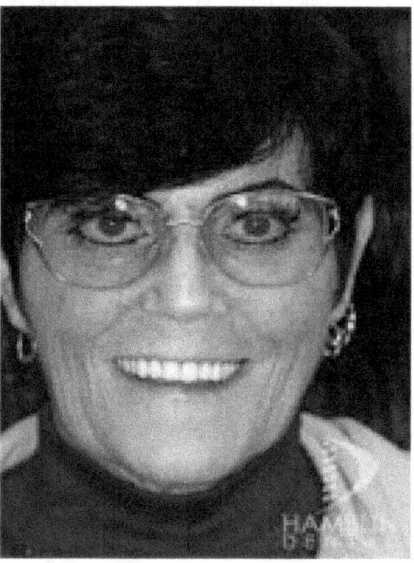

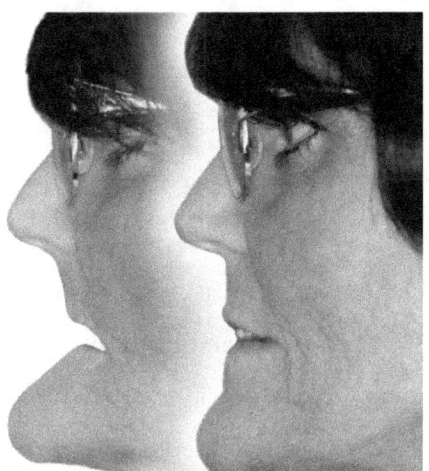

One way Dental implants can improve your smile is with a virtual facelift. Hybrid dentures can make you look younger by replacing the vertical height lost from missing teeth. *Implant dentures* lift a sunken-in facial structure, supporting the face for a more youthful look while improving the vertical dimension and profile.

A Hidden Benefit of Implant Dentures

Another way Dental implants lift your smile is by keeping your jawbone healthy. Jawbone deterioration often accompanies tooth loss. Without a connective tooth root, your jawbone no longer receives the chewing stimulation your jaw needs for your body to send nutrients. As a result, the jawbone will begin to shrink, adding to the collapsed mouth look. The dental implants used in hybrid dentures restore the needed chewing stimulation, keeping your jawbone healthy and strong.

Dental Implants

Dental implants are now, the standard of care for tooth replacement, improving the dental health of millions of people with missing teeth. A dental implant refers to the post placed in the bone. The abutment is the extension attached to the implant, supporting the crown. Work performed by a laboratory is just as crucial as the work by the surgeon/ restorative dentist for long term success.

Laboratory cost can be significant for quality prosthetic work whether it is a crown, bridge, veneer, or denture. Quality laboratory work requires angulation and form of the abutment and artistic porcelain work for a crown that looks good with careful attention to details, communication with the dentist, precision fit, accurate margins, custom, and functions well.

All of this laboratory work takes time and professional expertise, which is why a quality laboratory commonly charges $225 to $350 for the abutment and another $250 to $300 for the crown fabrication. The longevity and success of implant-supported crowns depend on accurate and high-quality work. Non-fitting components and poor quality materials will cause crowns or dental implants to fail.

Yes, dental implants improve patient's quality of life from the standpoint of being able to eat healthier foods, and there are some studies done that show patients who do not have teeth live on average I think it is five years less than people who do have teeth. It is probably even more than that. I cannot remember the exact study, but it is at least five years shortened life span when you do not have your teeth.

With dentures, because you are not eating healthy foods, you are not able to chew things properly. Your digestion starts with your teeth so if you are not able to chew properly, your whole digestive system is thrown off. You want the dentures to look natural, so the goal is functionality. With cosmetic dentistry, porcelain veneers or porcelain crowns and also dental implants should look natural in addition to beautiful and function properly.

Age is not a factor when your quality of life is what's at stake. I have treated a patient from California, who was ninety plus years of age. She swam every day, had dentures, and lived a very active lifestyle.

She wanted her teeth fixed so she could eat and go out with her friends. She wanted to swim and not have her teeth fall out in the pool. It was so rewarding to help her obtain nice solid implanted teeth that fit well and did not fall out.

Another patient from Lake Powell is one hundred and three years of age. Ten years ago she had many teeth problems, and we fixed her teeth. She was probably ninety-three years of age at the time. She still comes into the dental office and gets her teeth cleaned and checked. She is doing great, and her smile is fantastic.

I was the team dentist for the Oakland A's who are located in California. About ten to fifteen years ago, one of the most notable players needed dental implants. I performed the surgery on a Friday afternoon and told him to follow a liquid diet and to not chew anything all weekend. On Monday, he came back into the office, and he was bleeding profusely. Very concerned, I asked him how long he had been bleeding. He said that he went out for pizza after surgery and the stitches tore open, and he had been bleeding every since. He was a professional athlete and had bled a lot. We re-sutured the area, and the bleeding stopped. The point is that it is so important to follow the home care instructions we give you.

You can still get gum disease with implants. The dental implants cannot decay, but the gums can deteriorate causing gum disease. The gums must be maintained and kept clean.

Many patients have had root canal after root canal, and the teeth keep breaking off. The teeth need to be extracted, and the patient needs a bridge. The two adjacent teeth need to be ground down to put the bridge. An option for this patient is to take out a tooth, put an implant in without grinding the two adjacent teeth down.

If the tooth goes bad or breaks off at the gum line, it is not restorable. We take the tooth out and put a dental implant in and put the temporary crown all in one day. Sometimes, the patient elects to try and save the tooth. The dentist does a buildup of a crown that might work for a week or might work for a year but is no long term solution. The dental implant will be there two decades or more than likely the rest of the patient's life.

In my own mouth, I had a root canal tooth that went bad and had to be removed. I elected to go to Philadelphia to a dental implant specialist whom I trusted. He placed my dental implant, and that was ten years ago. That tooth is probably my most solid tooth, I had two teeth taken out and was missing a tooth for a couple of months. I gained sympathy for patients who are just missing just one tooth let alone all of their teeth. It is a struggle to eat solid food.

Ten years ago I had a patient come in who worked as a Certified Nursing Assistant. She did not make much money, had severe periodontal disease with infection in her gums and bone. Her teeth were loose, and she could not eat anything. Of course, that was affecting her health. We took out all the infected teeth, put in dental implants and gave her a nice solid fixed bridge that is attached to her dental implants. For her, it was a choice between a new truck or new teeth.

She chose new teeth and just like other patients that we have treated, never regretted that decision.

Another patient came down from Wyoming and after a phone call, I felt she might be a little unstable and was hesitant to treat her. She was thirty-four-year-old single mom with a fourteen-year-old daughter. She ran a dry cleaning business. A dental professional in Wyoming had removed all her teeth and provided her with dentures. The dentures would not stay in her mouth so every time she talked they fell out.

She said she was almost suicidal, and I was concerned about the difficulty of the situation. She turned out to be our best missionary for implant dentistry. We put in dental implants in the top jaw and the lower jaw. She now has porcelain teeth that look beautiful, and she can chew whatever she wants. The work we did turned her life around. Her business succeeded, and her daughter is in college. Her social life is fantastic, and the confidence behind her smile changed her life.

"No Pain, No Bleeding, No Sutures"

Yes, this statement is possible, but a few things need to occur. First of all, there is always some discomfort with a dental implant placement, although mild in most cases. Surgery without bleeding or sutures means that a dental implant was placed without an incision and gum tissue flap. This is entirely possible. However, here's the catch: The team must use a CT-scan for 3-D workup and fabrication of a unique guide to aid the surgeon for precise implant positioning.

I have used this technique many times with great success. It does add to the cost, though, often by as much as $750 to $1000. It is well worth the additional charge if there are multiple implants, compromised bone anatomy, and a need for great accuracy in difficult cases.

Without the 3D planning, placing implants requires a "blind" implant placement that is difficult and challenging, even in the hands of the most skilled surgeon. Even if there is bleeding, it usually stops in a few hours and sutures fall out in few days. I do not recommend compromising dental implant positioning and accuracy to avoid slight bleeding and sutures.

Implants have a more than 98 percent success rate when performed by the right dentist that uses quality implants that are customized by a laboratory.

As far as improving the quality of life, I had a patient fly in from West Virginia. Her dad was a coal miner, and she was about my age. She had dentures since she was 14 years old! Emotionally, she wanted solid, secure teeth, and she did not want anything that resembled dentures. Sometimes fake gum tissue is required to make the final prosthesis, cosmetically acceptable. The longer you have been wearing dentures, the more likely it is that you will need some acrylic or porcelain that resembles gum tissue.

She did not want any pink acrylic, she wanted all of her teeth to look the best that they could, but she did not want anything to resemble dentures. She did not want any pink acrylic on there, and when she smiled she wanted it to look great. She was the choir director and was embarrassed having her dentures falling out in front of her choir.

I put in the dental implants and now she has teeth that stay in and are solid. She was so thrilled with the results because she could hit the high notes and open her mouth wide, with total confidence that her teeth were solid as a rock! Her quality of life was dramatically improved with dental implants. This is just another example of my rewarding career improving the quality of life. Psychologically, she was a changed person. I was so happy for her.

I consistently hear my patients say "I wish I had done this years ago." It is a significant investment for the patient, you know they make that investment, but also every time they come in afterward they bring in home baked cookies or apricots off their tree or tomatoes from the garden. They are just grateful for what I've done for them, it is emotionally rewarding for me, and I love doing dental implants. I change people's lives for the better.

Zirconia Dental Implants

Originally the first dental implants (the 1980's) had two parts: the fixture (which goes screwed into the bone) and the abutment (where the prosthetic crown is cemented).The improvements in new ceramic materials made it possible in 2000 to have the abutment part made of ceramic. This material was commonly known to be more tissue friendly than titanium.

In 2005, the CeraRoot full ceramic implant (fixture and abutment in one body/part) was introduced into the European market and in 2011 accepted by the FDA to be used in U.S. dental clinics. The main advantage of a one-piece zirconia implant is that it has no prosthetic connections, where bacteria can grow, and therefore have better gum health. Another big advantage is that the implant is 100% white. This means that no metal will ever be visible when smiling or communicating with other people. One of the problems of zirconia implants in the past is that did not come as two parts (Implant and Abutment). This means that if the patient's bone is angled in a different direction than the alignment of the teeth (this is very common), and you could not correct the angle by using an angled abutment. There are companies now that make two piece zirconia implants which can be used to correct the angle of the bone.

My opinion is that zirconia implants have come a long way, but my first choice is the tested and proven Titanium implants.

Throughout the decades, the materials that have been used for the dental treatments have been made with metal. The main reason was to give mechanical strength and therefore augment the longevity of the treatment. Over time, the scientific research contributed enormously to the improvement of the ceramic's mechanical strength. In the beginning, ceramics were introduced into the patient's mouth because of its fabulous esthetic properties.

Stop Smoking

Dental implant surgery success rates go down into the seventy percent range with heavy smokers. Healthy non-smoking individuals, regardless of age, who have dental implants, experience a success rate of ninety-five to ninety-seven percent.

I have a patient who is a plumber and a heavy smoker. He had upper and lower dentures he could not stand and wanted fixed porcelain teeth. He was honest about the fact he smoked two packs of cigarettes a day. I told him he needed to stop smoking before he could have dental implants. He claimed he had quit smoking, but he did not quit. A year later he had a couple of dental implants fail, and we realized he was still smoking a lot. The year after that he had a few more dental implants fail, and the situation turned into a big waste of money and time for both him and me.

Dental implants are a big investment, so if you are not willing to quit smoking, you will waste your time and money. If you are a heavy smoker, *do not* have the procedure done.

How do I take care and maintain the health of my Dental Implants?

Caring for implants is simple and no more difficult than the care that should be given to natural teeth. This includes **DAILY** hygiene using a prescribed anti-bacterial agent and proper brushing techniques as instructed along with regular check-ups and x-rays as recommended by the doctor. Although, implants are not susceptible to decay like natural teeth, they are vulnerable to poor hygiene that will cause bacterial build-up around the gum line which can lead to infection, bone loss, and eventual failure of the implants. Regular hygiene is a must to maintain the health of implants and natural teeth.

Equally important is a well-balanced bite which can be insured by proper loading of the implants (aspects involved in placing the teeth on the implants is my job) as well as regular follow-up visits to maintain a balanced bite (patient's job). Implants are stronger in the bone than natural teeth. However, like natural teeth, implants are susceptible to uneven chewing forces which over a period can cause bone loss and possibly eventual loss of the implant(s).

Lifetime health maintenance is also an important factor in the long-term care of dental implants. Just as serious health problems can affect natural teeth so can they affect implants?

Bone Grafting

The gold standard with bone grafting is using your own bone. The next best thing is cadaver bone. I have been using cadaver bone for years with no complications. Sometimes, in particular for religious reasons, the patient does not want cadaver bone, and I will use synthetic bone grafting. The synthetic bone graft does not work as well as your bone or cadaver bone, but it is an option.

What is TMJ?

Migraines are sometimes caused by Temporomandibular Joint (TMJ) dysfunction. Patients are treated with a night guard called an NTI. The NTI is very simple to make, and it is installed in the mouth to relieve pressure on the muscles in the TMJ. The patients rave about how they have not felt that good in years. The patient must have been clenching and grinding which was giving them headaches. The "*wow*" factor is the lack of a migraine headache.

Holistic Dentistry

Holistic dentistry also called biological dentistry, alternative dentistry, unconventional dentistry, or biocompatible dentistry. Holistic dentistry emphasizes approaches to dental care said to consider dental health in the context of the patient's entire physical as well as emotional or spiritual health in some cases. Although the holistic dental community is in its practices and approaches, common threads include strong opposition to the use mercury/

amalgam materials in dental fillings, non-surgical approaches to gum disease, and the belief that root canals may endanger the systemic health of the patient through the spread of trapped dental bacteria to the body. Many dentists who use these terms also regard water fluoridation unfavorably.

Many practices and opinions among alternative dentists are criticized as not being evidence-based by the mainstream dental community and skeptics of alternative medicine in general. Generally speaking, such dentists charge far more for the same dental treatment compared to mainstream dentists, as they consider themselves to be providing special care.

Metal-free dental implants have several benefits:

- Zirconia has become popular as a desirable implant material because it interacts well with the natural gum and bone, making it biocompatible.

- Metal-free implants are biological dental implants, meaning they are a more holistic option for those interested in treatments that support total health.

- For cosmetic reasons, zirconia is a better choice. Titanium dental implants can cause a dark line around the gum. Zirconia is a more natural color, eliminating this effect.

Because of the increase in interest in holistic dentistry and metal-free treatments, zirconia dental implants are gaining in popularity. For patients who suffer from sensitivity to titanium, metal-free dental implants offer an alternative.

Whether you are concerned about potential complications presented by having metals in the mouth or if you are simply looking for a more natural result, ceramic dental implants are an alternative to titanium dental implants. Holistic dentists tend to offer ceramic dental implants to their patients precisely because they support a metal-free philosophy. However, from my experience, and the complications associated with ceramic implants, my first choice is still titanium. Maybe technology will improve for ceramic implants.

Impact on Sex Life

Moreover, lastly, according to a recent study, being fitted with dental implants can have a positive effect on your sex life. The study, compared the impact of social and sexual activities by 102 adults between the ages of 35-65 years, before and after being fitted with dental implants, against people equipped with conventional dentures only. The research revealed that the subjects equipped with implant-retained dentures experienced a greater increase in comfort felt during kissing and sexual activity over a two month compared to those with normal dentures.

Patients reported that conventional dentures often became loose during activities such as kissing, eating and speaking, resulting in both embarrassment and discomfort. Of those participants who experienced loose dentures when kissing, more than 80% felt uneasy when kissing, and 70% felt awkward when engaged in sexual relations.

My patients are continuously overjoyed by their new smiles. Their only regret is that they did not get dental implants earlier. I love making their smile beautiful!

4

DENTAL OFFICE TEAM

Are the team members friendly, compassionate and effective?

The dental team like the dental hygienist, dental assistant, surgical assistant, and the entire front office staff are considered a team and should be friendly and compassionate. The dental team treats you with respect and is clear with financial arrangements. The team members that are hands on should be experienced, gentle and caring. An appointment should be scheduled with the doctor, and there should be no charge for the consultation. You will get to meet the staff and team members and see what the office is like and how they operate.

A Google or Yelp review will give you an idea, but you must do a physical visit to determine if you are comfortable. Seeing how clean the office is, meeting the team members and determining if the people in the front office handling the billing are professional. The front office handles the insurance and billing, and it should be clear before you start treatment how the cost will be billed.

There will be no surprises when it comes to the cost of the procedure. You should be aware exactly what the insurance is going to cover but if the fee is $10,000 that means $10,000. If your insurance covers eight hundred or two thousand dollars, it is a contract between you and the insurance company. Our estimate is going to stay the same regardless of what the insurance pays.

My surgical assistant is probably one of the best that I have ever worked with. She is so good that I am tempted, that if I need an implant or a crown, that I would almost let her do it. I would not do that, but she is so good it is tempting. She is almost competent enough to be a dentist, and I trust her with my patients because I know she does quality work. She makes the temporaries and works with the patients and makes them comfortable.

The office needs to be clear with the patients that they are to show up on time because it could delay our schedule for other patients. Everyone hates the waiting room when his or her appointment is delayed. If you show up half an hour late, we are half an hour behind schedule for the next patient.   Being punctual is very important for a dental office to run smoothly.

Experience of the Doctor

How experienced is the Doctor?

I've been placing implants for over 27 years. I graduated from Baylor College of Dentistry in 1985. Back in 1985, the dental school said dental implants were voodoo, witchcraft, and don't work. I started attending dental implant courses in addition to dental school. I even traveled out of state to go to dental implant specialists to learn about dental implants. I was fascinated with dental implants even before they were accepted by the dental community.

I set up a private practice in the San Francisco Bay Area in 1985, in Danville California. I was the team dentist for the Oakland A's baseball team for about ten years. I started to get very interested in cosmetic dentistry during this time frame. Many professional athletes and famous people wanted to look like Hollywood stars. Non-celebrity people like you and I wanted to look better too, and so I got trained and started doing a lot of cosmetic dentistry.

What should you look for in a cosmetic dentist?

When looking for a cosmetic dentist, especially one specializing in dental implants, you should look at their experience.

- How long have they've been placing dental implants?

- How many dental implants have they placed?

- Ask for referral information from a few former patients they have treated including names and numbers. When you call these former patients be sure and ask them if they were happy with the results.

- Ask for before and after pictures of the cosmetic dentistry, they have performed. Notice if the work looks natural and at the same time enhances the patient's face and makes them more beautiful.

I've been placing dental implants for 27 years and even on the extreme or more complicated cases that are very expensive and require substantial costs out of pocket, the patient has been happy with the result. Many patients have lived with dentures, crooked or missing teeth for years and are so glad to have a more beautiful smile. Most patients wish they had done the cosmetic procedure years before. The patient comments consist of "I've been living with these dentures for ten years", "I've been living with these crooked and broken, missing teeth for years.", "I wish I had done this years ago" or "I wish I knew about this earlier."

Like I said earlier when I was in dental school I was intrigued by dental implants. I started going to dental conferences outside of dental school in my spare time. In 1987, I started research and training with Jerry Niznick, who was considered the dental implant master of the time. I have placed implants for almost 30 years. However, it was not until about ten years ago that I started focusing on just dental implants.

I took one year off, and I went all around the United States and Canada. I studied with Thomas Balshi (that is who placed my implant) in Philadelphia, Joe Vassos in Edmonton Canada, Karl Mish, and many other dental implant experts. I trained in all aspects of dental implant surgery. From bone grafting, sinus augmentation to the new 'all on four." I went into their offices and observed them placing dental implants. I also observed how they handled surgery, and I did surgery too. I spent an entire year so that I could specialize in dental implants.

When I am not in my office, I mentor and teach other dentists in the western United States. My unique method for dental implant surgery, dental sedation and aesthetic dentistry are the best in the industry and sought after continuously. We offer non-invasive dental implant surgery training in our True Dentistry office, in Las Vegas. Dentists come from all over to attend our courses.

In my own mouth, I had a root canal tooth that went bad and had to be removed. I elected to go to Tom Balshi in Philadelphia. Tom is one of my mentors, whom I trusted, and he placed my dental implant. He did that work over ten years ago, and that tooth is probably my most solid tooth. I have had two teeth taken out and was missing a tooth for a couple of months. I have sympathy for patients missing one tooth let alone many teeth, especially a group of teeth on one side. Every time you eat something like nuts or chips it feels like your gum is getting stabbed with a knife.

I had a patient a few years ago who was in his nineties, and he was in a rest home. The patient had dentures and could not wear them. Therefore, the food they fed him was put through a blender to create soft, baby food, consistency. He could not stand it.

The man was in great shape for 90 and golfed every week for the last 65 years with his three brothers. All four of them served in World War II. At 90 plus years of age, my patient knew what he wanted. At this age, you might think he would not want to spend the money and get beautiful, solid teeth. However, he decided to get dental implants.

After healing, he began to eat corn on the cob, steak, and other solid foods. He got out of the rest home now, and he is eating anything he wants. He is grateful for his new, solid, secure implanted teeth. He may only live ten more years, but his quality of life for those ten years is better because he has teeth that he can chew and smile with. He can eat healthier fruits and vegetables and digest them much better.

The man has more confidence, can go out in public, and not worry about his teeth falling out.His quality of life was significantly increased, and he was very glad even at 90 years old he made a major investment in his health and his smile.

Past Patient Reviews

Are the Dentist's former patients happy with their care?

You can research a dentist on Google or Yelp and read reviews about that dentist. You can gather information through these reviews. The dentist could have a few negative, but you want 80 or 90 percent of the reviews to be positive, and possibly the comments saying "wow! This doctor was gentle, and the implant looks perfect!" Visit the dentist's website for private endorsements from patients, including testimonials. Sometimes a dentist may give out a former patient's phone number or email (with prior consent from that patient) so you can reach out to those people to call and talk and hear about their experience.

If you already have a dentist you like and trust, that explains all fees and procedures before starting treatment, who practices pain-free dentistry and who never makes you wait to be seen, then please disregard this invitation to join our practice. I know that once our patients have experienced that with us, it is difficult for them to leave us, even if they've moved out of the country.

Selecting a dentist can be a difficult task so here is some information that will help you choose a dentist that's right for you. Our dental office was created so you can experience friendly, gentle Dentistry that produces proven results – a great smile and healthy teeth for life.

Question 1: How do I know I'll like my experience if I come to your office?

As a patient, you will notice a difference the moment you step into our state-of-the-art facilities, designed for your comfort. Many of our patients have remarked to us what friendly, upbeat offices we have. We take personal pride in being an office that our patients like to come to. If you have not been to a dentist in a long while, you can be assured of not being embarrassed or scolded.

We know it can be hard to come in even though you know you should. We will not make it any harder. We work to make it easier so you can feel relieved about that! We work with you individually to help you get the right kind of dental care that looks good, feels good, and helps keep your teeth for a lifetime.

At our dental office, we have the latest technology available in equipment, materials, and technologies so you can have not only excellent dental health but also a great smile. You'll enjoy a friendly, upbeat atmosphere of open communication.

We answer your questions and work to understand your concerns. We also offer something that is very unusual in a dental office which is the "Cannot Go Wrong" 1st Dental Visit –GUARANTEED or It is FREE. We offer a special offer that prevents you from making a mistake in choosing your dental office. It is simply this: if after the 1st visit initial clinical examination, you decide we are not right for each other, you can leave and pay nothing

Question 2: How do I know you are a good Dentist?

I have a passionate commitment to giving you quality dentistry that looks good and feels good. Good dentistry comes as a result of the combination of education, ongoing professional postdoctoral training and teaching, talent, experience, and the commitment to doing it right.

I pride myself on providing a friendly, caring chair-side manner. I pay attention to the details that ensure your care is as thorough and as gentle as possible. I love a challenging dental situation, and I love to make people be able to have that beautiful smile. I provide a broad range of diagnostic and treatment methods to determine the best for your situation.

Question 3: Do you offer all the Dental services that I need or could need?

The short answer is "yes" but at our office, we offer all the dental services that you'll ever need. We are a full-service dental practice, and I can help you with all the routine services you would expect, along with the ones that you do not commonly see in most dental offices.

Among the routine services we offer are examinations, cleanings, check- ups, conservative gum treatment, fillings, laser diagnostics, advanced x-rays and computerized dental diagnostics, root canals, crowns, bridges, removable partial dentures, and cosmetic dentures.

Also, we offer the following services:

- Cosmetic Dentistry Services- Smile makeover based on com- puter assisted Smile design to give you a look you've always wanted.

- Super-safe removal of Mercury fillings

- Super-Strong tooth-colored materials, so teeth do not look gray or dark at the gum line, giving natural looking teeth

- Full cosmetic consultation for challenging, difficult situations such as restoring smiling and chewing to normal

- Bad Breath Evaluation and Treatment

- Advanced digital x-rays-greatly reduces radiation to about a day at the beach

- Dental Implant Therapy to replace missing teeth and rebuild smiles, performing all aspects of the treatment, surgery, and restoration since 1987

- Gum Therapy which includes using dental lasers, plastic surgery for your gums to make them look right, regenerative surgery using bone grafts to rebuild missing bone, specialized antibiotics to treat resistant gum disease

- Customized Cosmetic Dentures with porcelain teeth that look stunning and natural

- Intra-oral video and digital cameras that let you see what we see when we look into your mouth

- FDA Approved Migraine Headache Prevention- that is 77% effective in reducing migraine headaches

- Wisdom tooth removal

Our patients say they like the fact that they do not get sent all over town for their services.

Question 4: Do you make appointment scheduling, fees, billing, and insurance easy for me?

The dental office should recognize the importance of being able to get appointments and having a flexible schedule. We also know how valuable time is, and that is why you will never wait to be seen. Our office is different from most offices because we do not overbook appointments. In return, we ask that our patients come on time and not change appointments.

We help you understand the fees, billing and insurance so you can be comfortable financially, too. We work to make fees affordable while helping maximize your insurance coverage. We deal with thousands of plans and file for you helping you win in dealing with insurance companies. Dental insurance, while not a pay-all, can be a real help in paying for maintenance and basic dental care.

Question 5: Does the dentist have before and after photos of his current patients?

The doctor should have before and after pictures of patients for your review. If you are looking at the photos, make sure the cosmetic improvement looks natural. Do the teeth have natural grooves or valleys in them and when that patient smiles do the teeth reflect light naturally? If the new teeth look opaque, like Chiclets, flat, fake with no translucency, then you may want to look elsewhere.

If you take a flashlight hold it behind your teeth, you're going to see the light at varying degrees come through your tooth, and so translucency is natural at the incisal edge. Adding just those components makes a world of difference in making the tooth look more natural.

So the anatomy of the teeth and the translucency both make a replacement or a prosthetic tooth look much more natural and undetectable.

I love to show before and after pictures of my patients. It makes me so happy to help people have a beautiful smile. I want to show off my work and help others.

Here's What One of Our Patients Had to Say about Her Experience

"I met Becky, Dr. Hamblin's Patient Coordinator, over the phone after calling numerous doctors throughout the Salt Lake Valley. It was because of her warm and caring personality that came through the phone that I first chose to make my appointment with Dr. Hamblin.

Over the phone, I explained my dire situation. I had many dental procedures throughout my life. Just about everything. However, I found myself in a nightmare. I had no teeth at all. In 45 minutes a local dentist removed all of my remaining upper and lower teeth. I was not old enough to need dentures. I was desperate.

My first meeting with Dr. Hamblin was very comfortable physically and emotionally as well. He took the time to go over every procedure he felt I would qualify for. In the end, I decided to go with Implants. "Teeth in a Day" sounded so farfetched, but I am proof of it! After a couple more consults, a complete step by step procedure list, and cost evaluation, I went in for my 'surgery', the actual implants.

To my disbelief, it was the definition of quick and painless. I do not remember any of the actual time in the chair, and my recovery was one-third of what my healing was after my previous extractions. I had teeth! I could smile! I could go back out in public and most of all I could once again join my only daughter in her life outside our home.

*The impact of having such a drastic situation of having zero teeth, I mean NO teeth, just gums, was for me, life threatening. I was on the edge of considering suicide. All I had ever wanted was something so small, just to be able to have my picture taken with my beautiful daughter. Sounds so small, but it was impossible before becoming a patient of Hamblin Dental. I was back to work in 2 days and did not even finish my pain management medication. I did not need it. **THERE WAS NO PAIN!!!!!!!!** Let me say that again; THERE WAS NO PAIN! I would not have believed that if 100 Heavenly Angels came before me and said that. I knew dental procedures, and this one was going to hurt. Wrong!*

Somehow Dr. Hamblin and his incredible staff of professionals have perfected everything about implants. Everything from the impressive location of his office to the warm nature of Becky, on to the very competent and friendly assistants for the doc, but mostly to Dr. Hamblin's up to the minute current education, skill, drive, knowledge, incredible human nature, and desires to help others reclaim their lives.

Every step of the way I felt no anxiety and no unforeseen problems have come up. The cost was sizable, but when in return, I get to talk, smile, & interact with others. I get to live again. How do you put a price on that? I have my life again. For years, I had been depressed over my appearance and wouldn't interact socially with anyone except immediate family.

Now I have that interaction back in my life. So if you can qualify for the financial, have the need, and want the BEST, then Dr. Hamblin is the one to go. If my before picture is included in this testimony, it is scary, more to me than anyone. I know this, and this was one reason I felt I had to agree to show it and was asked for my testimony. I think I have to be one of his full mouth restorations! If he can help me, he can help you. It is such a drastic difference, so only click on it if you are not weak at heart! Drastic Picture Warning! These words are just a summary of what I could go on and on about. Really, how in the world can I put into words what it feels like to have another chance to live life? It is not easy. So if anyone has any questions ask! Your answers are right here with Dr. Scott Hamblin."

-Julie H. - Wyoming

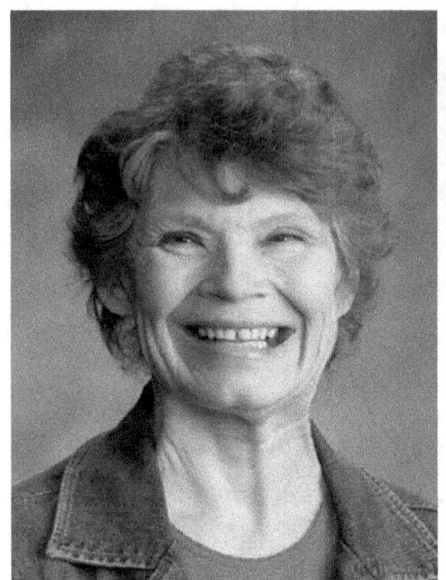
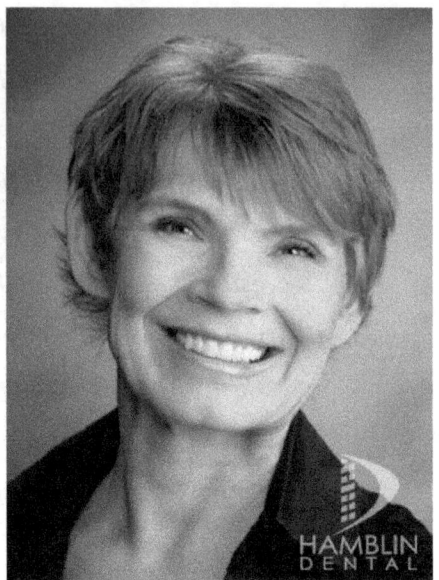
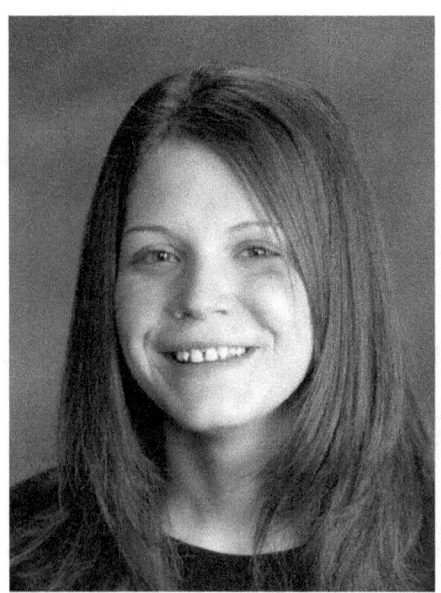
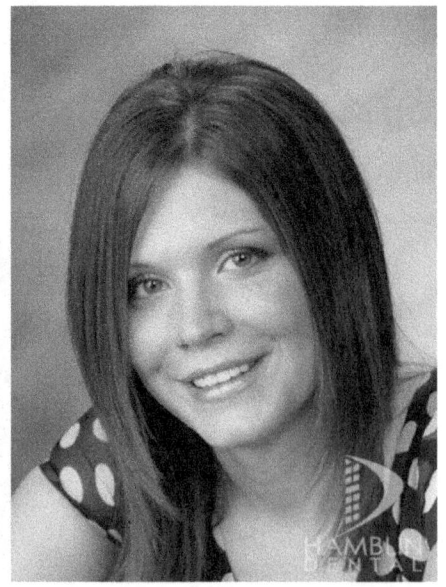

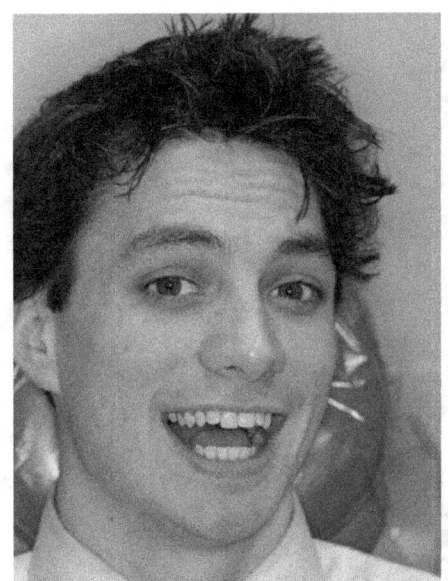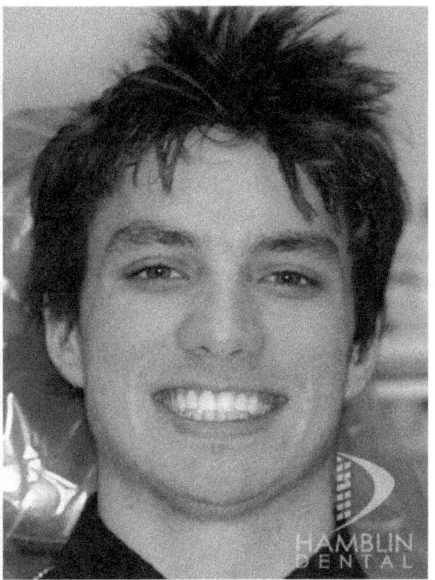

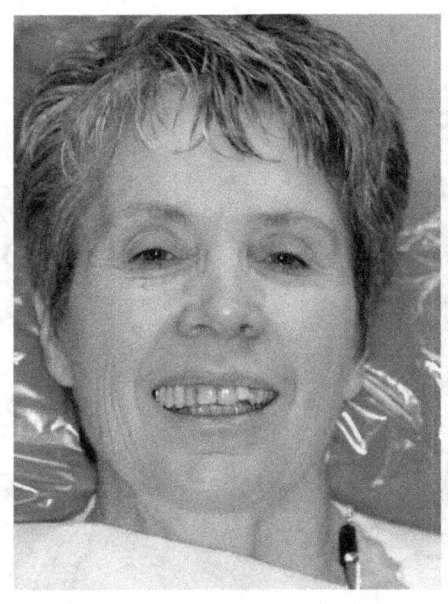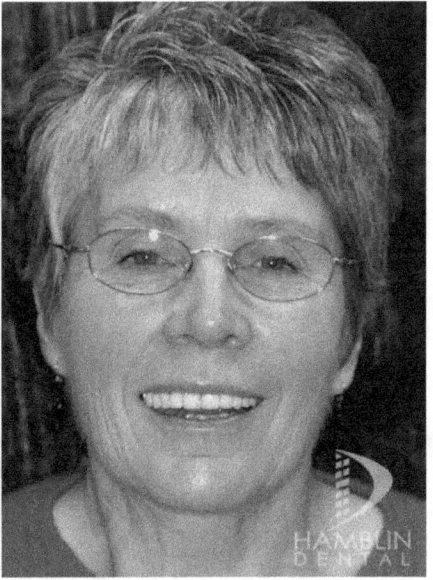

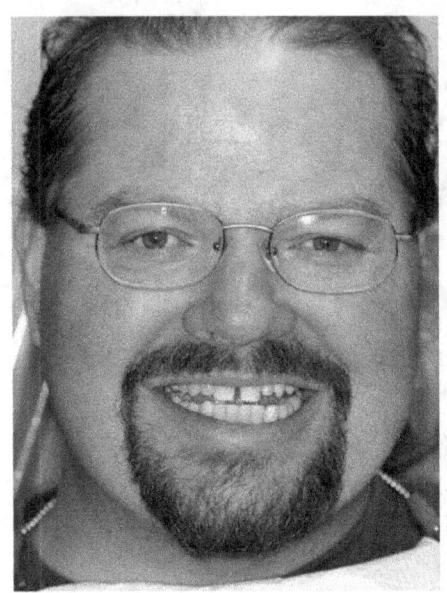
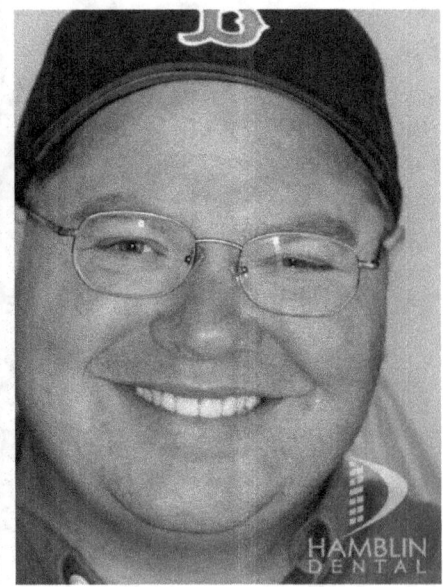
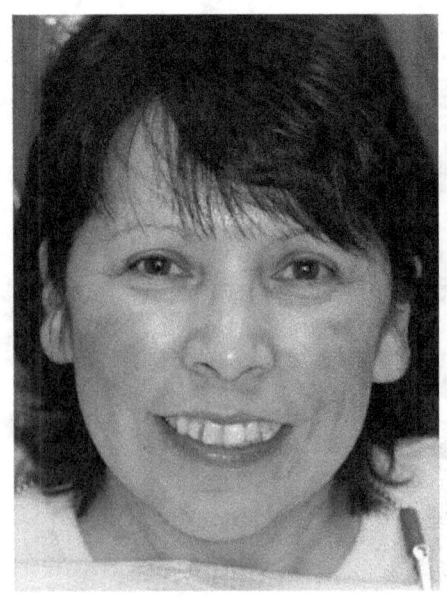
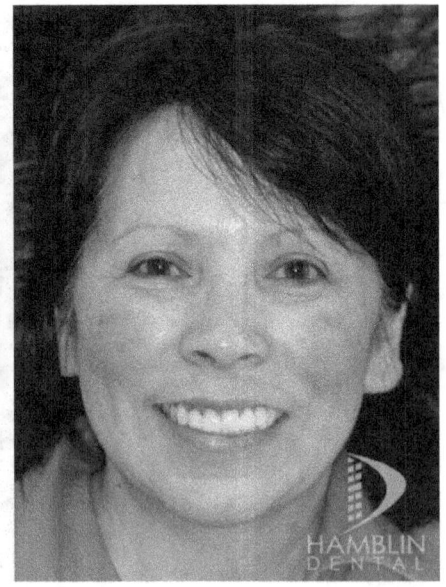

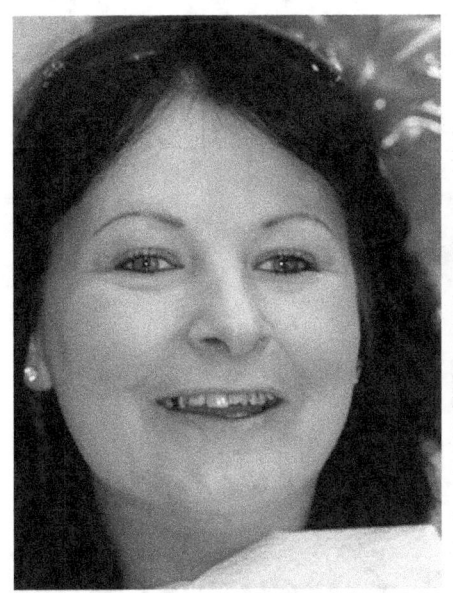 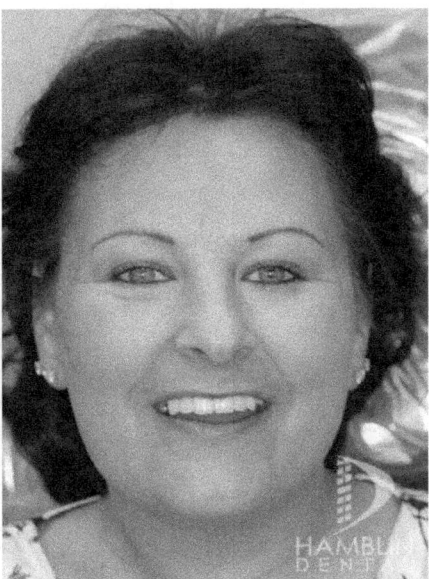

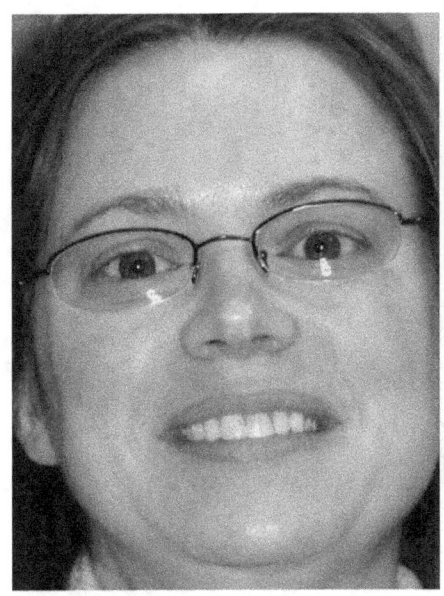 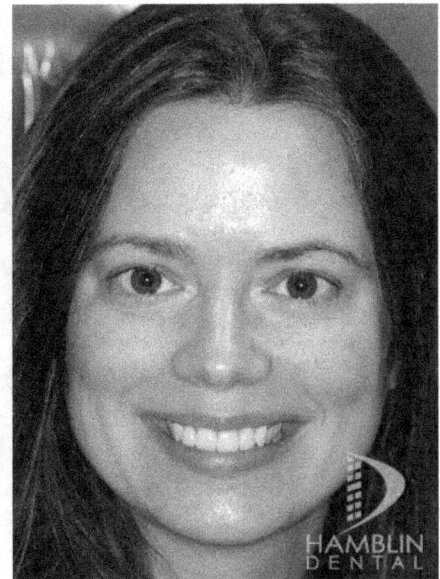

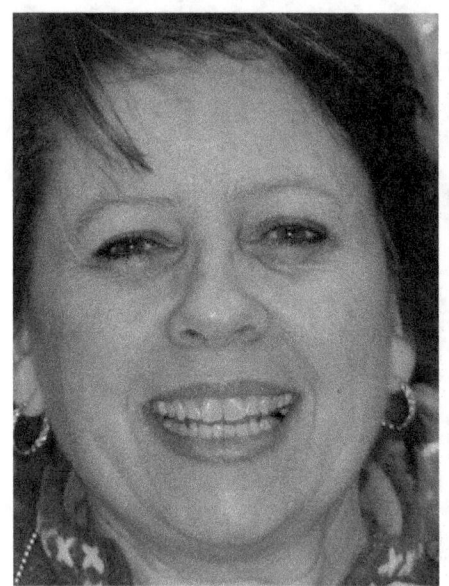
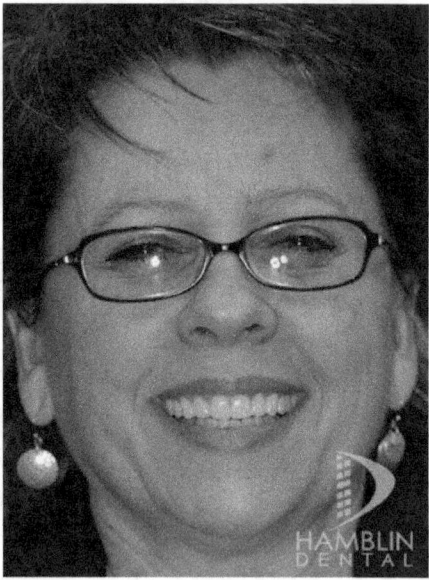
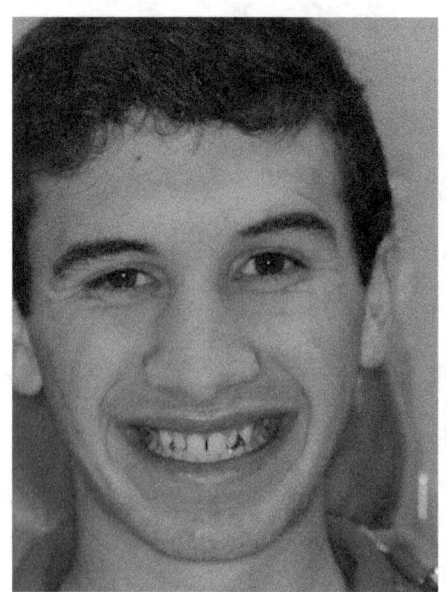
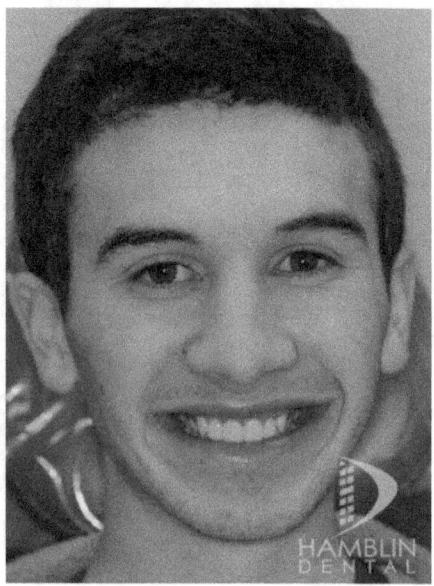

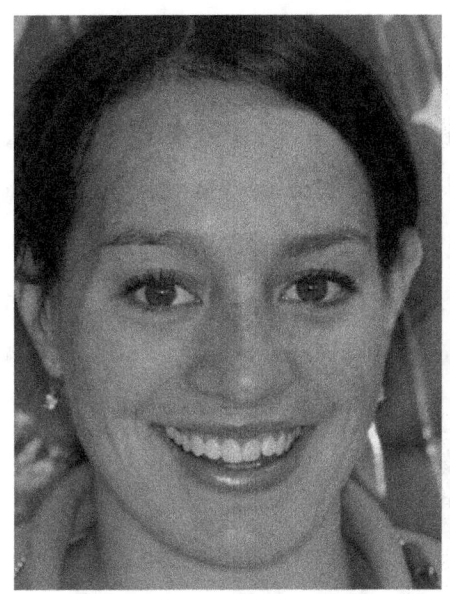
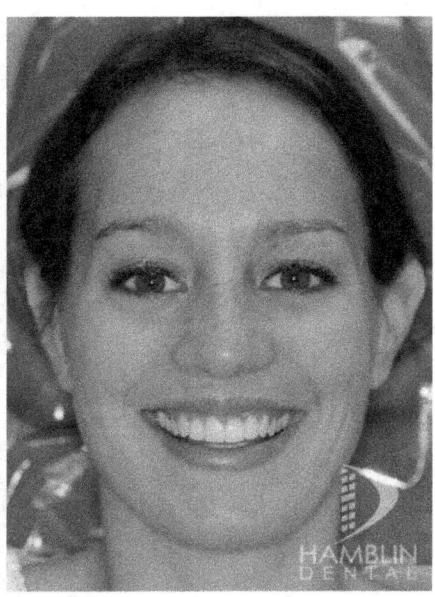
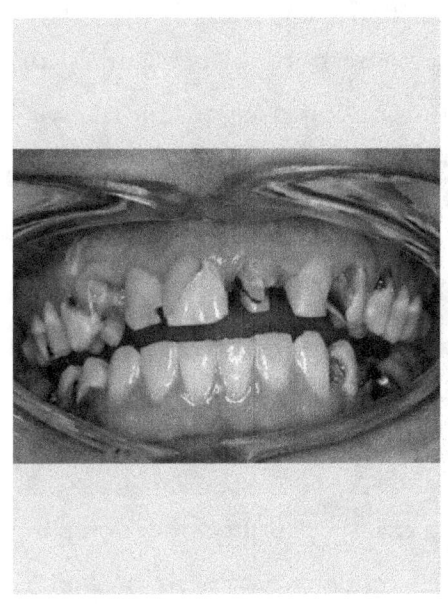
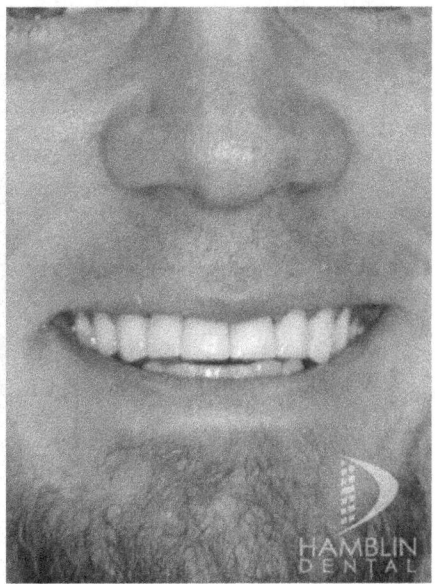

Treatment Options

Does the dentist offer you options in treatment (i.e. Good, Better, Best)?

The old rule "If it is too good to be true, it probably is" applies to dentistry too. When looking for tooth replacement options, do not fall victim to misleading marketing tactics. Do your research. Ask the right questions. Know what you are getting. It is a lifetime investment and shouldn't be taken lightly.

Personalized care vs. going to a big box dental chain.

I have an opinion about "chain" clinics. I believe they have a cookie cutter approach to every patient. In my experience, there should be multiple treatment options. I have seen patients for a second opinion after going to Clear Choice (Big Box Chain store). Every patient I have seen was given the exact same treatment plan, regardless of the condition of their teeth! The only option given was the "All on 4" surgery and hybrid screw retained the acrylic denture. Acrylic/resin fixed dentures tend to take on odor and stains fairly soon.

One patient that came to us after going to one of these clinics felt suspicious when the clinic pushed them to start treatment immediately. I feel that with big decisions like this, you should feel comfortable and be given ample time to discuss things with your family.

I am not certain as to the clinics exact fees or how they compare to my fees for implant surgery, the temporary prosthesis, or the final prosthesis, but I do know that my patients consistently tell me that they 'wished they did this years ago.' From my experience, patients have felt the value they have received from us was well worth it.

I know that no matter where you go to have dental implant surgery, the fee you will be quoted will probably be twice what you expected. You need to decide several things; if the improved quality of life is worth it, if the doctor is experienced, and if you are getting the best VALUE and the best care for YOU.

The "chain" clinic may provide an estimate that is just the cost per implant. If the treatment plan is too aggressive, the cost of the surgical phase and the prosthetic phase could be more than what is best for you and your budget. It is always in your best interest to go to a dentist you trust, who is more conservative in their treatment, and gives you options.

The "All on 4" technique was developed by Nobel Biocare and Paulo Malo from Portugal. Nobel is a reputable dental implant company, and Dr. Malo is one of the most knowledgeable dentists I have met. I agree with his concern about helping patients by avoiding extensive bone grafting and trying to keep the costs affordable.

However, I also like the final prosthesis (set of teeth) to be made of porcelain fused to gold or porcelain fused to titanium, or even porcelain to zirconia. These options look very natural, involve less maintenance, and don't pick up bad odors and stains over time as an acrylic prosthesis will. Regardless of which final prosthesis you opt for (acrylic or porcelain) be sure your dentist is highly experienced and willing to stand behind his or her work.

Some patients ask me if age is a factor, or "Should I do this at my age?" I think the question you have to ask yourself is, "Can I live with these dentures or these teeth for even five more years?" To be a good dental implant candidate, you do need to be in good general health but age is not a factor. It is a quality of life issue for most of our patients.

Our patients want to be able to chew and smile without having unsightly or painful teeth. One thing I will say about being a good dental implant candidate, you have to promise to take immaculate care of your new teeth. If you cannot do that, there is no reason to go on with treatment. It would just be a waste of your time and money and mine as well. If you are in general good health, and you promise to take immaculate care of your new teeth, you qualify as a candidate for dental implants in our office, regardless of age.

Smoking increases the risk of failure in dental implants. Smokers are 2 1/2 times more likely to have implant failure than a non-smoker. Don't even think about having dental implants placed by me if you plan on staying a heavy smoker.

For dental implants to be able to be placed in your jawbone there needs to be enough bone present. If you lack good quality and quantity of bone, there are bone grafting procedures that may be able to give you back enough bone to now place dental implants. I try to avoid bone grafting, but when it is in the patient's best interest, I will always make the recommendation that is best for you, or what I would want for myself.

We have some of the most competitive fees in the country. In fact, we have had many patients fly in from California, Florida, and Georgia and save tens of thousands of dollars. To give you some guidelines, though, you are looking at from $1000 -$2500 for the surgical fee for a single dental implant. That is assuming that no bone grafting or special procedures are required. Placing the crown or false tooth is an additional $1000- $2500.

If you are having a complete set of teeth placed with dental implants, there is more variation possible because there are so many different ways to tackle that problem. For example, a simple snap-on denture for the lower teeth, retained by two dental implants, can cost from $2500-$7000. If you want to go first class with your new smile, you could spend $50,000- $100,000 PER JAW, for complete replacement of every tooth.

If you are considering dental implants, ClearChoice dental implant centers might appeal to you. ClearChoice Dental Implant Centers can be found in many cities now. You have seen their TV ads, radio, billboards and large full-page newspaper ads. They are very aggressive in advertising. See what they recommend and then see us, and you will see the difference for yourself.

Implants have also significantly impacted dental economics with increasing number of dental practices and companies offering their services and products. To gain market share, many dental practices advertise dental implants in the newspaper, with mailers, or on the

Internet, offering incentives to attract potential patients to their offices.

If these offers sound too good to be true, they usually are.

Dental Tourism

People will go to Mexico or Costa Rica on vacation for these extensive dental treatments to save money on a costly procedure like dental implants. Dental implants are a significant investment for the patient, and so some patients think they are going to save money and go to these clinics out of the country.

People think they are saving money but then come back to the United States and the work has to be redone or replaced. There is a lot to be said about the ability to go into an office if something goes wrong rather than fly out of the country. We have many patients that fly in from Florida, West Virginia, Texas and California. Many patients from my California practice still come to see me in Utah. So, why travel out of the country?

The service may be cheaper initially but when you have to get the procedure redone because of defective materials or defective surgical techniques that cause the implants to fail, was money saved? I have seen patients, that went out of the country, have loose dental implants or worse, an infection around the implants.

5

ONE DOCTOR, ONE OFFICE, ONE DAY

Is the Surgeon capable of performing all related procedures?

Many patients want to find a doctor who can provide all the services related to dental implants in one office. Finding a dental office that can provide all implant related services can be difficult, but why wouldn't you want that? Many times patients are confused because they are only getting a cost estimate for one part of the procedure and not the whole procedure. It feels like a sales pitch that has hidden items.

Find an office that is one doctor, one office and one day. I mean one day to do the whole procedure which involves taking out the teeth, putting the dental implants in, doing the bone grafting and putting a solid set of temporary teeth in. The entire procedure is done all in one day. So someone who comes in with dentures allows us to put in 4 to 6 implants, and the patient leaves the office with a fixed temporary bridge that's solid. It is not the final bridge, but it is a temporary bridge that's not a denture, it is not a set of removable teeth so, therefore, one doctor, one office, one day.

With an implant, the lower jaw takes about three months for the implants to integrate with the bone and the upper jaw about 4-6 months, so anywhere from three to six months you'd come back and get your permanent set of teeth or your permanent tooth. It is convenient to go to one office where the costs are clear. You do not have to navigate Google Maps for three different doctor offices and take time off of work, or time away from doing what you love.

I hear quite often that our patients appreciate being able to come to one place. If something goes wrong with the implant and the oral surgeon placed it, the dentist put the tooth in, and there are two or three other doctors involved, who is responsible? Who is going to stand behind their work?

At our office, we stand behind our work because we are doing the extraction the bone grafting the implant and the cosmetic tooth afterward.

When looking for a cosmetic and implant dentist you want to find someone who is comfortable and experienced in providing all of those services.

I offer *"Teeth in a Day"* which is a new scientifically proven break-through in dental implants that allow denture wearers and those suffering from other severe dental problems to have new solid teeth implanted in **ONE** appointment. Imagine having a restored freedom to smile, laugh at will, and enjoy a quality of life that you felt was gone forever. My *"Teeth in a Day"* procedure gets you back to living life to the fullest in as little time as possible.

I have treated patients, who like you, may have one or several of the following problems:

- Extreme fear of the dentist

- Missing teeth

- Teeth that are a complete mess

- Ongoing tooth loss

- Dating, and sex life embarrassment

- Dentures that don't work

- Loss of self-esteem

- The feeling of being incomplete

- Problems eating and speaking

- Worsening medical conditions because of poor nutrition

- Inadequate digestion of food

All of these problems can be solved with my special methods of dentistry. *"Teeth in a Day"* is the fastest way to get from one of life's most frustrating conditions back on the road to dental health and wellness again.

Every dental patient benefits from *"Teeth in a Day"* technology. Even those who are not ideal candidates for the procedure still have reduced treatment time for EVERY dental implant procedure. Procedures that once took months to complete *can now be condensed into a matter of hours or days* thanks to advanced CT scans, 3D modeling, and computer aided surgery and design. I am proud to be a pioneering doctor bringing these advancements to the general public and for the benefit of my patients.

There is one major problem with this technique. This problem involves how long one waits before deciding to move forward with this type of care because the longer you put off a consultation and treatment, the greater your chances are of not being eligible for this new "teeth in a day" procedure; quite literally the clock is ticking. If you want to benefit from these latest advances, the very best thing you can do for yourself is come in for a 15-minute complimentary consultation to discuss your options as fast as you possibly can.

Due to the very high demand for this new "teeth in a day" procedure, my teaching obligations and because my team and I ensure that each patient is cared for in a proper manner, my team and I have a limited number of consultation appointments and actual treatment times available. The bottom line is that the sooner you call, the better your chances at getting one of these limited times.

To let you see how life changing dental implant technology is, I've included photographs (color photos can be seen on our website www.DentalImplantsUtah.com) other patients who at one time felt that they 'couldn't be fixed' but now are living every minute of life to the fullest again. Take one look and you can dramatically see how their lives have completely changed after experiencing care by our team of dental professionals.

The patient went from thinking there was no hope to finding out that they still had workable and permanent solutions to get back the smile that the ravages of time or accidents took away.

It is very likely that someone you know **desperately** needs to know about this revolutionary new technique and that there is still hope for them. I am asking that you please share this book with them. You can feel satisfaction knowing you have helped change their life for the better too.

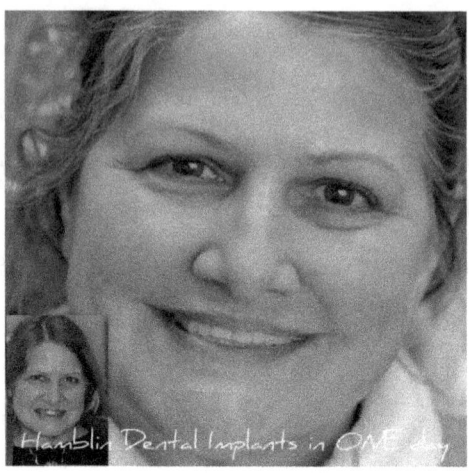

Good News: Who Wants to Live Longer?

One of the things we've learned just in the past few years from new medical studies is that you may *live up to 10 years longer* just by having a healthy mouth! Patients that have diseased mouths DIE sooner and have more heart attacks and strokes. Getting your dental health back extends your years.

Bad News: Dental problems get bigger

With this new scientific information, we know that as your dental problems get **bigger,** and your number of options shrink, your risk for dentally related heart attacks and strokes keeps growing. The sooner you get back your dental health, the sooner you can begin to reduce these dental risks to your health for years to come.

Many people who use to have missing, failing teeth or loose/ill-fitting dentures are now telling me how they are eating and enjoying the foods that they have not been able to eat in so long. They are **tasting**

the foods they are eating and don't have to mess with denture adhesives through the miracle of their new dental implants. In this book, you will find many instances of evidence showing serious health problems that are associated with bad oral hygiene.

In the past, when someone lost a tooth or many teeth, the most common approach to solving that dental problem was to put in a partial or full denture. However, with the advancements in dentistry, you can have stronger, fully restored teeth while giving you the appearance of secure natural looking teeth with dental implants.

If you are a candidate for our Revolutionary *"Teeth in a Day"* procedure the actual extractions, implant surgery and replacement teeth are all placed in ONE DAY. You will come in for a consultation to see if you are a candidate for this new procedure. We obtain a cat-scan that takes 20 seconds, not the 30-minute ones done in the hospital. That is all you've got to do.

The next step is we use that cat-scan and plan out your surgery on a very sophisticated software/hardware application. A very precise surgical guide is made specifically for your surgery. We evaluate everything and then have our on-site lab artistically make your new teeth that will be fixed solidly in your mouth on the day of your procedure.

The implants are placed and a "conversion prosthesis" is placed. The conversion prosthesis is only temporary but is nevertheless fixed solidly in your mouth the same day the implants are placed. You will need to return to our office about three months later to fabricate the final porcelain teeth. Doing implant surgery the traditional way can take much longer (approx. 9-18-months) depending on the type of implants and quantity of bone in which the implants are placed. Not everyone is a candidate for *"Teeth in One Day"*.

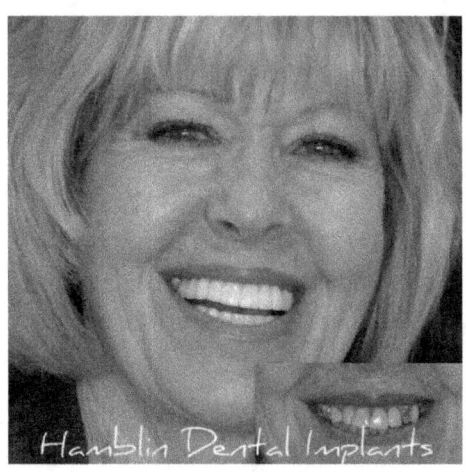

Want to Stay Out of the Nursing Home? Then Get Your Teeth Fixed

Another recent study showed that your odds of being in a nursing home are much higher if you wear dentures because of denture related health problems that help rob you of your independence. Things are usually so bad in your mouth at that point that you cannot wear your dentures and even if you could the nursing staff often loses them.

All this means that the denture wearer in the nursing home suffers ever worsening medical problems from poor nutrition and lack of attention from the poorly paid and overworked staff who could care less. Finally, the most unfortunate thing is that the *last memories left* behind for your grandchildren are of a favorite grandparent *without any teeth*. Thanks to **"Teeth in a Day"** and my other dental implant advancements, I am happy to say that my patients have fewer chances of experiencing these undesirable possibilities.

Conclusion: *Why Wait?*

The most important thing I can tell you is that the longer you put off seeking a solution to your problems, not only will it become ever more difficult, complicated, painful and expensive to find a workable solution BUT there will come a point when there is no solution. I've seen patients in the past few months that made what they thought were rational decisions during the recent years. They decided to put things off because of all the problems they see in the newspaper or on TV and missed their last chance for a solution and are now *miserable*. It breaks my heart every time I tell a patient that even if they had acted a few months ago, I could have taken them from being a "disaster" to a happy patient with a strong, healthy bite and beautiful smile.

Right now, no matter how bad you think your problems are (even if you think they are already pretty bad), just wait a little longer and they are guaranteed to get far worse. I am sharing these hard facts with you, so you understand that the time to reclaim your dental health is right now. If you act now, you are likely to have many more ways to get back your dental health; including *"Teeth in a Day"* technology.

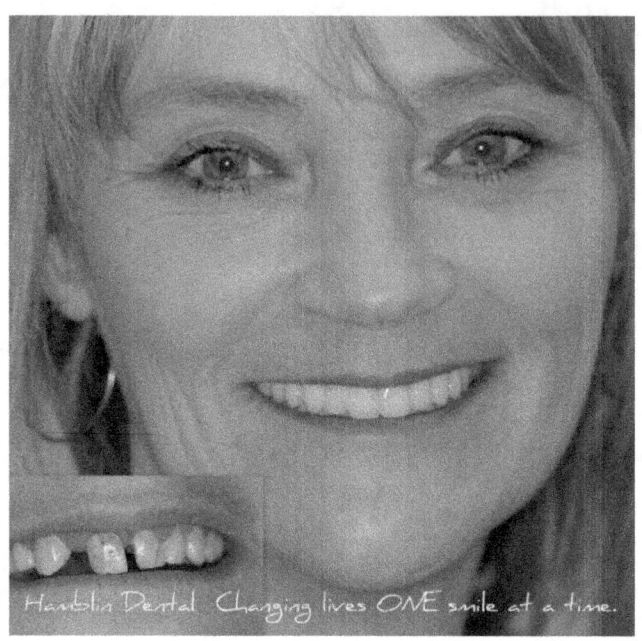

The Best Day is Today

I have discussed many positive items in this book but even knowing all of these things, why would any patient put things off while knowing that "Teeth in a Day" and other new advancements in dental implants are possible? Here's why. It is human nature to resist stubbornly change, even when it will profoundly benefit your whole life and health. Outwardly, of course, you make excuses that attempt to justify why it is not the time to take action to regain your dental health just yet.

The most common excuse is "the time is not quite right." Someday, you insist, "When all the pieces of my life fit perfectly together, I'll be in a better position to take action, get back my ability to eat comfortably and smile again." You are only fooling yourself with that phrase. It is like thinking that someday your train will arrive at this picture perfect station at the end of the line, and then you can do all of the things you have meant to get done. That day never arrives UNLESS you take action.

The reason that most patients get caught up in this delusion is they do not know "how" to take the first step. **Your first step is a 15 minute "talking" consultation** in my office to discuss briefly the benefit of "Teeth in a Day" and other advanced options for your individual situation. Yes, making the appointment for that first visit is hard BUT not impossible. Moreover, of course, the 15 minute "talking" consultation is complimentary to find out what new technique best provides a solution for you.

Please don't miss the opportunity to take advantage of the latest in treatment options AND most importantly, don't allow yourself to become a patient that even I could not help. Keep your hope alive.

Out Of Town Guests

I am fortunate to have a loyal following of visitors from all over. Whether you're from Salt Lake City, Las Vegas, or out of state we'll make your appointment as convenient as possible. It is our pleasure to accommodate our out-of-town guests by assisting with travel arrangements, hotel accommodations, restaurant reservations and ground transportation. Imagine, come to Salt Lake or Las Vegas for a few days of shopping, skiing or relaxation and go home with a spectacular new smile!

Preoperative Instructions

Implant Patients

It is essential that we have as much information including preliminary models, films, scans, etc. completed at your initial visit and give the best dental care.

- Digital photographs: full face serious and full face smiling, lip retraction, occlusal view

- Panorex film

- Study models and bite registration

- CAT Scan, Upper and Lower Jaws

- Desired shade for temporary prosthesis, if applicable

Smile Makeovers

If your plan is to have a cosmetic (dental implant) smile makeover, it is essential that we have the following information:

- Digital photographs: full face serious and smiling, full face lip retraction, occlusal view

- Panorex film

- Study models and bite registration

Preoperative Clearance

Implant and Sedation

Certain patients may require preoperative clearance for dental implants. This is determined on an individual basis.

Preoperative Financial Arrangements

Financial arrangements and any required deposits must be made prior to your visit.

Required Paperwork

Call our office and we will mail the required forms to you, or you can now download all necessary forms.

www.dentalimplantsutah.com/contact-info/patient-forms

If possible, complete the forms and send them to us before your visit.

Treatment Options

After carefully and thoroughly reviewing the necessary information, the dental team and I will design treatment options specific for you here in Sandy Utah. Together, you can decide which procedures will be best for you and for your lifestyle.

Send Digital Photos, X-rays, Study Models, Bite registrations and CAT Scans to our Dental Care Coordinator:

10011 South Centennial Parkway Suite 540

Sandy, UT 84070

801-255-7645

mysaltlakedentist@gmail.com

or in Las Vegas

True Dentistry

9061 W. Post Road

Las Vegas, NV 89148

Phone: 702.434.4800

The Day Of Your Surgery

Implant Patients

Your surgery will be performed in a surgical room located within our office. We encourage patients to travel with a family member or a close friend who can assist in your postoperative care. It is a standard of care to have someone with you for 12 hours following your surgery. It is advised that you have someone assist you following oral sedation.

Smile Makeovers

It is advised that you have someone assist you following oral sedation.

Postoperative Care

Implant Patients

Plan to stay in Salt Lake City or Las Vegas from 3-7 days after surgery depending on which procedures you have performed. This will be decided during your phone conference.

Your Return Home

When you go home, it is important that you follow all of the printed instructions for your recovery. Some procedures may need a follow-up visit. Please include this in your planning.

6

COMFORT MEASURES

Will you be treated gently and will you feel comfortable?

The other thing you want to do when you go into a dental office for a consultation with the doctor is how comfortable you are in the office, in particular, the reception area. Is the physical building comfortable, clean and inviting? Some offices have big TV screens and some patients like that. Some doctors like that.

I do not have big TV screens and make it a point to have more of a personal connection with the patient. If the TV is always on, it feels like there is another person in the room and the patient and I have a difficult time understanding and listening to each other.. Our patients love the view of the Utah Mountains. In Utah, there are many weather changes with the seasons of fall, winter, spring, and summer. Our patients say it is soothing to have openness in the office.

We use memory foam for the dental chairs, so the patient is comfortable. We also offer oral sedation and/or laughing gas for your comfort.

What aids in pain management does the Doctor offer?

The doctor should offer painless injections, topical anesthetic, and gentle, caring hands.

Is sedation offered?

Can you rest comfortably through the entire procedure?

With dental implants or any other extensive appointment, the dentist should offer sedation including oral sedation. The patient takes one little pill about one hour before their appointment. The patient is not completely out but doesn't remember being at the office. The patient is very comfortable, and the appointment goes smoothly.

If the patient wants to be completely out, the dentist can provide an anesthesiologist as part of his team to give IV sedation. It is hard to tell how gentle a dentist is until he/she has worked on you. During the exam when the dentist is looking in your mouth is he/she pulling and tugging on your cheek and shoving your head around or is he/she gentle and concerned about your comfort.

The dentist should place topical anesthetic, and let it work for about

3 minutes before giving the injection. Also, acupressure can help eliminate the sting of the needle. We use a compounding pharmacy to make our topical anesthetic. It is much stronger than you can just buy out of the dental supply catalogs and we leave that on for two to three minutes, and the injection is relatively painless. You are still going to feel a little bit of a pinch but it you know want to make sure that the doctor is capable of giving a painless injection.

If you have been terrified to go to the dentist or hate getting any dental work done, then you must read on. You can have an *enjoyable, pain-free, stress-free experience when you go to the dentist.*

25 years ago, I came across a very special procedure that only a small percentage of dentists are doing that has changed the lives of many patients because it allows anyone to get all the dental care he or she needs without any fear or pain, in one visit!

I saw men and women who had the most awful, fears and phobias from their old dentist. They left our office after their first visit saying that was the most pleasant and enjoyable experience they've ever had at "any" doctor's office.

I saw people completely fearful walking in, but within moments, they were as calm, relaxed, and pleasant as a sleeping baby. I heard stories from patients who suffered **their entire life in fear of even the slightest thought of needles,** or the smell, or sounds of the dental office, who were now more confident and entirely fearless. The best part was that they had healthier and more beautiful teeth than ever before, because of what occurred within a very short time of being in our office.

These people left the office feeling great and having a whole new view of going to the dentist. In fact, each and every one of them referred all their family and friends. I was so impressed that I *got trained in Sedation Dentistry Myself! Moreover, that was 25 years ago!*

It is strange how life is because now people of all ages come to see me and get the smile they've always dreamed of. We specialize in treating people who fear going to the dentist by using sedation dentistry.

Simply put, when you come to our office "you sleep while we treat" and you won't experience any pain at all. People come to me for conscious sedation if they have the following:

- Fear of needles

- Have had bad experiences in their past with a dentist or in a dental office

- Have dental phobias

- Toothaches or Headaches

- Suffer from TMJ syndrome

- Are in need of a crown or bridge

- Old silver fillings that need to be replaced,

- Had some SERIOUS tooth decay and it was affecting their

overall health

- Experience Low Self-Esteem or Poor Self Confidence

- Experience Constant Oral Pain

- Cannot get numb with anesthesia

- Want to sleep through their dental care using sedation dentistry,

- Alternatively, simply anyone who wants a dentist who will give an anxiety-free and practically pain-free experience while guaranteeing his work.

- Bad Breath

- Trouble eating certain foods

Many of my patients have tried different ways to alleviate their fear of going to the dentist with little or no success. They have searched for years, using hypnosis, meditation, and even going to therapy, but never did they think they could go to an office where Fear, Pain, and Anxiety are a thing of the past.

Their hopes and wishes for this type of dental experience seemed like just a dream until now. Now, I can do the same things my mentor showed me, without my patients having to go through any fear, pain, or anxiety!

Several times per day patients thank me for curing their fears and giving them a confident more attractive smile and curing ANY fear they had of going to the dentist. However, I cannot take the credit. **My confession is that** *I've never really "cured" anyone of anything, or performed any miracles.*

What I do is perform sedation dentistry that allows you to come in and sleep through your dental care. What's so great about this is that you can get four visits done in just 1, because you are sleeping. That means fewer trips into see us, less time away from work, and more time for fun and vacations.

My goal is to bring the most effective and most advanced treatments to my patients so they can look and feel better NOW…and feel better forever! Our team has put together a comprehensive program to target ALL aspects of your dental health to get you the results you'd like as quickly and easily as possible.

Oh yeah. My second confession is that I could not help as many people smile with more confidence and get dental care without the help of my team!

7

FEES AND CHARGES

Are the fees inclusive and completely clear?

When you are purchasing something that's designed to last, it makes sense to do some comparison shopping—especially if that something represents a significant investment.

This could apply to cars, appliances, jewelry, even dental implants. However, wait a second: There's something about dental implants that is not quite the same as the other three items.

When you buy a car, an appliance or a piece of jewelry, you are buying a product. Dental implants, however, aren't just products—what you are investing in is a set of procedures or a process, you are investing in the experience and artistry of the surgeon. So what's the big difference?

Product vs. Process

Think of it this way: If you are buying an appliance from a big-box store, the price might be the main concern. Once you get it home—provided it is the same model—it does not much matter where it came from. The same thing goes for cars and jewelry, although the seller's reputation for honesty and service is usually taken into account. Still, barring any problems, you get the thing you've paid for, and that is that.

Dentistry and Dental implants are different. Unlike a product that you take the way it comes, implants are better viewed as a means of achieving the desired goal: The replacement of missing or non-functioning teeth with new, fully-functional and great-looking prosthetic teeth. However, you do not just pick those teeth up off the shelf and put them on—instead, after a careful examination, you go through the exciting process of deciding what your new teeth should look like, having them expertly crafted and placed...and then seeing your smile transformed. I know I wouldn't shop around for the cheapest heart surgeon. I do not think that your oral health is that much different.

Steps Toward Your Goal

If the process of getting dental implants is like a stairway to a new smile, then you could look at each procedure as a single step. You'll finish every step before moving on to the next; altogether, they will get you to the top. However, the procedure performed at each step—from your initial evaluation to your final follow-up visit—should be handled expertly and completely. Moreover, that's where the difference between implant providers may become clear.

For example, a premier dental implant specialist should first offer a complete 3-D CAT scan of the jaw as part of the examination process. Only then can a comprehensive plan for the exact procedures an individual needs be developed. Next, any preparatory work, such as periodontal procedures or bone grafting, should be completed. When everything looks satisfactory, the implant procedure can begin: Teeth that cannot be saved are extracted, the right number of implants are placed at correct locations in the jaw, and a set of temporary teeth are attached to the implants. To reduce the number of separate visits, it may even be possible to perform tooth extractions, implant placement and temporary crowns in a one-day procedure.

An Investment in Quality

Dental implants represent a significant investment for many people. It is not just the physical materials that account for the cost: It is the time and effort taken at every step of the process, and the experience of the dental implant specialist and caring clinical team members. You can shop around for a low price...however, it's the standard of care that makes all the difference in your experience, and in the final result.

Every person is different. We all have a different anatomy, different issues, and different needs. When it is time to make an investment in yourself by getting dental implants, be sure to choose carefully from among your options. While price is a factor, it is not the only one to consider. Transforming your smile is not something you can do simply by buying a product ...however, viewed as a process; it should be a rewarding experience.

Yes, it is expensive to get back what you've lost...however, you really cannot afford not to......

The truth is that dentistry that permanently solves serious problems *is expensive.* However, this is one investment that will *pay dividends* to your physical and mental health and wellbeing 24 hours a day seven days a week forever. Moreover, if that is not enough, you will likely live to enjoy these benefits even longer. How many other things can you spend your valuable money on that comes close to delivering those same promises?

By now you probably realize that **you really cannot afford not to do this for yourself.** My team and I have moved mountains and found new financial options so you can get the care you need. We are **THE** experts at coming up with financial solutions for almost any patient that wants to get their care done correctly.

Payment options

Does the dentist offer multiple ways for you to afford the care you need?

Cost-effectiveness and Health Benefits of Traditional Dentures versus Dental Implants. I have **started a study that compares Dental Implants to Dentures.** "We are looking at the cost-effectiveness ratios, taking all costs into account, and we define the effectiveness as the patients' satisfaction with the treatment. In previous studies, we've seen that patients are significantly more satisfied with implanted teeth than with traditional dentures.

Dental implants are more costly in the short term, but they have a greater cost-effectiveness ratio, which means they are less costly in the long run. Dental implants are surgically placed into the bones of the jaws, which adheres to and holds them tightly in place. Conventional dentures, which are removable, can be less comfortable and less stable, making it harder to chew solid food.

When dentures do not fit well, patients have to eat mostly mushy food like stews and soups but with dental implants, edentulous people show improved nutrition since they can eat more fruits and vegetables.

I have high hopes for health coverage for dental implant care that will improve with studies like this. In 20 years of dental implant surgery, I have only had medical insurance pay for the patient's treatment once, and that patient was starving to death. After having his teeth removed (due to severe gum disease) and dentures made by another dentist in Arizona. He went from 195 pounds down to 135 pounds in about four months. He was unable to chew properly and gagged easily, constantly throwing up, causing digestive problems, and obviously, malnutrition.

We placed four dental implants and made an implanted denture which made it possible for him to chew and not gag and vomit. Within four months of having the implants placed, he was almost back to his normal healthy weight.

If we show that people with Dental implants are healthier and have a better quality of life and that conventional dentures are not much cheaper in the long run, because of greater replacement and adjustment costs, then perhaps insurance companies and the government may be more likely to consider funding for dental implants. Currently, Medicare only pays for conventional dentures, and only for people on welfare.

The Government and Insurance Companies are trying to maintain their budgets, and the last thing they want is to start paying more for treatment that they feel is cosmetic. What they do not realize is that dental implant treatment has an enormous impact on quality of life and health. Unless there are studies like this, the insurance companies will continue to deny benefits to deserving patients.

The research is part of a new, patient-centered trend in medicine, in which patients are actively involved in choosing their treatment, and changing it if they feel it is not working.

When you are using patient-based outcomes, you are not just giving them treatment and then putting them on some physiological testing equipment. You are asking them about how much pain they have, and how they feel about their quality of life. Patient preference can give a more realistic idea of the actual effectiveness of treatment.

Consultation

We take the time in consultation to make sure you fully understand every appropriate option at our offices. We teach you about the latest methods of correcting dental problems from missing teeth to cosmetic concerns and dental problems.

Safety

Our entire team is well versed in the state of the art sterilization techniques designed to ensure your safety. This includes gloves, face masks and a state of the art sterilization center. If this is an area of concern for you, just ask for a tour. You'll not only be impressed but reassured: your safety is a top priority.

Payment Options

Credit cards such as Visa, MasterCard, Discover and American Express and also 12-month interest-free plans offer unique payment options.

Insurance

Our office employs a "Treatment Coordinator" who is knowledgeable and experienced in processing dental insurance and arranging convenient financing. Bring your group policy information in with you and let us do the rest of your dental insurance and help you understand all your dental payment options.

8

WARRANTY

Does the dentist offer a warranty on the work?

As a patient, you should ask the doctor about the warranty or guarantee they offer on the dental implant as well as the whole procedure including the cosmetic dentistry and the crown. All of these items are tied together, and you want to be able to get treatment in case something goes wrong. A doctor should stand by his warranty.

A good warranty should be at least five years. If the porcelain crown chips or breaks or part of the porcelain bridge breaks then, we repair that at no charge for the first five years. A dental implant has been around for at least 30years, and I've been placing them for 27 years. If the dental implant fails, it is usually in the first three to six months when the body either rejected or accepts it. If a failure of a dental implant occurs then, you want to make sure the doctor is going to put another one back in at no charge.

There is not a hundred percent success rate, but dental implants rarely fail after six months. The failure rate is practically zero unless the patient did not come back for cleanings, or did not maintain the teeth by following home care and maintenance instructions. The dentist should provide clear instruction for care to keep the warranty in place.

The patient should be clear on proper home care including, flossing, brushing, water pic, antimicrobial rinses, eating a healthy diet, avoiding chewing on ice etc., and not smoking. If the patient is following the instructions and coming every six months for checkups and cleanings, then the dental implants should last decades.

Even with dental implants the patient can still get gum disease if the patient does not maintain their oral hygiene. Make sure you come in every 6 months for cleanings and checkups to keep your warranty in effect.

9

YOU WILL LOOK 10 YEARS YOUNGER!

Dental Implants assist you in looking and feeling younger because they prevent bone loss. By preventing bone loss that would normally occur with the loss of teeth, your facial structures remain normal and intact. The chances of wrinkling and the look of old age before your time is less likely. Implants prevent the bone loss that would normally occur with the loss of teeth.

In other words, every day that you continue to wear dentures or have missing teeth, you are experiencing bone loss, which makes you look much older than you have to. By using dental implants **your facial**

structures and jaw remain strong, healthy, and intact.

This is especially important when all of the teeth are missing because the lower one-third of the face *collapses* if implants are not placed to preserve the bone.

1. **Overall quality of life is enhanced with replacement teeth that look, feel and function more like natural teeth.** You will look younger and more attractive which allows you to be even more confident and enjoy smiling, laughing, and talking with others.

2. **You can now live longer because you'll get to eat better and prevent malnutrition or stomach problems!** Fresh Vegetables, corn, and fruits are back on the menu! You can now eat the foods you like. Also, since your chewing is improved, your digestion will be even better!

3. **More Confidence in social situations.** Most of our patients love their new implants, because of their improved appearance, function, comfort, and health. When you go out in public, you will never have to cover your mouth with your hand, or put off eating out of fear of a denture popping out or gagging you. Also, the improved appearance of your new smile will have people giving you compliments galore.

4. **Allows you to relax and not have to worry about your dentures moving around, popping out, or gagging you.** You'll never worry about your dentures flying out when you laugh, sneeze, cough, or when you eat. Implants are so securely attached that the fear of them falling out will be eliminated! Like I said before, these will feel like they are your natural teeth.

5. **Your mouth will be restored as closely as possible to its natural state.** By replacing the entire tooth, as well as the tooth root, it is possible to replicate the function of natural teeth, with a strong, stable foundation that allows comfortable biting and chewing. Also, nothing in the mouth looks or feels false or artificial!

6. **Increases the amount of enjoyment you get out of eating.** You will be able to **taste foods more fully.** Wearing an upper denture can prevent someone from tasting food, as the roof of the mouth is covered. With implant supported replacement teeth, it is not necessary to cover the roof of the mouth, so you can truly enjoy the taste of foods.

7. **Improves overall oral health and decrease the risk of oral**

cancer and heart disease. It is much easier to care for implants of any kind versus dentures. Your chances of bacteria buildup and gum disease decrease when you have implants.

8. **Eliminate Denture Adhesives FOREVER!** Since implant supported teeth are securely attached to the implants, there is no need for messy dentures adhesives. (do a google search of new studies showing serious health problems associated with denture adhesives)

9. **Your other teeth will not be affected because of missing teeth.** Since replacing missing teeth with implant supported crowns and bridges do not involve grinding or drilling the adjacent natural teeth, they are not compromised or damaged. For example, when you wear a partial denture, you have clamps that hook onto adjacent teeth, which put pressure on them that causes them to loosen and come out. Bridges require grinding down of the adjacent teeth so that the bridge can be cemented on them. This tooth structure can never be replaced, and the long-term health of these teeth is compromised.

The benefits of implants far outweigh the benefits of wearing dentures or living with missing teeth.

10

MOST FREQUENTLY ASKED QUESTIONS

Below is a list of the most commonly asked questions that we receive from people just like yourself? Some may not apply to you. Just skip those and go to the next one that does.

Q: Am I A Candidate For Dental Implant Treatment?

A: Almost everyone who is missing one or more teeth and in general good health is a candidate for dental implant treatment. A few medical conditions that can undermine the success of implant treatment, such as uncontrolled diabetes. However, few conditions would keep someone from having implant treatment altogether.

Quality and quantity of available bone for implant placement is more often a factor in qualifying for dental implants than medical conditions. However, even people who have lost a significant amount of bone can qualify for dental implant treatment with additional procedures to add bone or create new bone. Advances in this type of treatment have made it possible for thousands of patients who would not previously have been considered candidates to have successful implant procedures.

Q: How Painful Is Getting Dental Implants?

A: Most of our patients report that they feel very little, if any, pain during the procedure. In fact, many patients do not have to use any pain pills. Your decision to use implants will help you to avoid much pain and discomfort in the long term.

Besides, given the overall health care benefits, you should not deny yourself proper treatment out of fear of pain. As with any medical or dental procedure, your attending doctor, the dentist, is equipped to provide you with appropriate treatment, including any pain medicines you need.

Finally, to make sure you are comfortable when you leave our office, you'll get a prescription if necessary. Our goal is to give you stronger, more comfortable teeth, without experiencing pain or discomfort!

Q: Will I Need To Have One Implant Placed For Each Tooth That Is Missing?

A: No. In fact, it is possible to replace all of the lower teeth with a denture that is supported by only four implants. On the other hand, sometimes it might work to your advantage to replace your back teeth with an implant for each tooth to provide additional strength.

Q: How Long Do Implants Last?

A: Most research has shown that implants have been successful for over 30 years. However, our goal is to make them, so they last a life-time. This is much improved from dentures, which last about five years, and/or bridges where the expected time of use is between 7-10 years.

Q: Do You Offer Any Warranty?

A: Yes. Even though dental implants have over a 95% success rate, there is still a very small chance that they will integrate completely with the jawbone. When this occurs, new implants are placed, and the success rates for the replacement implants are even higher.

If an implant needs to be replaced, which is very rare, it usually happens before the prosthetic teeth are even started. When we replace the implants, we remove the implant that the body rejected and placed a new one for FREE. The only thing you need to do is make sure you come in for your regularly scheduled preventive visits so that we can keep your implants, gums, and teeth healthy, which will prevent most possible problems. Long-term maintenance of your new teeth depends on which type of teeth you selected. Acrylic teeth need to be removed (only by us), and your implants and gums cleaned. Then the acrylic teeth are placed back in by us. This may need to be performed every 3-4 years. For porcelain to titanium teeth, they usually don't need to be removed by us to clean them professionally.

Q: How Do I Know If I am Too Old For Implants?

A: Great question. Your overall health and your desire to improve the quality of life are much more important things to look at, than your age. We currently have patients from 20 years old to 98 years old.

Q. Will I have to go without teeth at any time during my Dental Implant Treatment?

A. In the majority of cases, patients will always have temporary teeth to wear during treatment and in most instances the temporaries can be worn throughout the treatment period. There are those cases, however, where temporaries are not needed or where temporaries should not be worn for a few days after surgery. This aspect of treatment is discussed during consultation and treatment planning so that the patient knows what is expected regarding "temporaries."

Q: What is the Cost of Implant Treatment?

A: Many people call and ask us, "How much is one implant going to cost?" While I wish it were that simple. The only way to determine actual cost is by coming in for a consultation and examination to find out if you have bone loss, or if you'll need one, two, or more implants.

Q: How Much Will Dental Implant, Cosmetic, And "Sleep" Dentistry Cost?

My unique method of Dentistry means that for almost every patient there is still hope and several options to choose from. After you choose one of my exclusive options to solve your problems permanently, you'll feel great about yourself having regained the normal chewing, long-lasting beauty, and comfort that you deserve.

Dentistry that works well and lasts *IS* expensive; just like everything else in life these days. We wish it were not true, but it simply is. The good news is that you will have a hard time naming another investment you can make in yourself that provides the dividends of a pleasing smile and comfortable chewing 24 hours a day, seven days a week.

Prospective patients often ask, "What's a ballpark on cost?" Attempting to give you an exact range of costs for your specific situation over the phone is impossible since your problems and needs are unique just to you. I could have a "one size fits all fee", but some patients would greatly underpay, and others would greatly overpay. Hardly anyone would think that was fair! I devised a complete dental, physical examination just for the purpose to eliminate guessing so you can get your "one of a kind" options with complete costs and length of time for your treatment.

If You Have No Teeth, Are Wearing Dentures, Or All Your Natural Teeth Are "Shot:"

New teeth can be attached to implants and are either non-removable or removable from the implants. Removable is less complex and thus less costly. Non-removable are the best option and are more costly because of the complexity. The lowest cost dental implant options start at $5500-$8,000 per jaw IF you already have a perfect denture and perfect bone structure under the denture (a VERY rare occurrence). For the newest technologies such as *"Teeth in a Day"*, treatment averages $25,000-35,000 per jaw. In the most extreme cases, where patients waited for a very long time to seek a solution, care can surpass $40,000 PER jaw (also a rare occurrence).

If You Are Missing One Or Two Teeth:

For single teeth, a dental implant can range in cost from $2900-$6500 depending on whether it is "easy" or a highly complicated front of the mouth tooth. The tooth at the front of the mouth is very difficult to conceal and may appear unnatural to others. Also, cost depends on whether you select *"Teeth in a Day"* technology.

If your Natural Teeth Are Worn Down And "Tired" From The Aging Process And/or, You Are Missing Some Or Many Of Your Natural Teeth.

You probably need a reconstruction using implants and crowns/veneers on your natural teeth. What's a reconstruction you ask? Think of it as a remodel for your mouth and just like remodeling a hundred-year-old house, reconstructions are complicated scenarios; all the more reason you need one of a kind answers like I offer. Reconstructions range from $16,000-$30,000 per jaw.

SLEEP DENTISTRY FOR THE FEARFUL

The cost for sleep dentistry (where you <u>"sleep" through the visit</u>) if no dental implants are involved, starts at $1800-$5,000 and goes up based on how severe your problems and your specific wants for your situation.

Because my time is very limited (he devotes some of his time to teaching other doctors how to be better at the very same type of dentistry you are pursuing!), membership in his practice is limited. Your next step is to apply and have a complete dental, physical examination so you no longer guess about what your care will cost. The sooner you do, the sooner you'll be on your way to comfortable chewing and a smile you'll be proud of.

About medical and dental insurance: Even though the latest dental technologies are considered medically necessary and are scientifically proven, dental plan coverage to rescue the worst dental disaster patient hardly touches what is needed to get you back to the healthy life of eating and self-confidence you deserve. The objective of the insurance company is to give you the <u>cheapest</u> possible care. This seldom provides for anything beyond basic generic emergency based treatment which is not what my method of dentistry is all about.

Here are some ways that our other patients managed their costs and got their care done:

- Using cash (5%), credit (2.9%) and senior (5%) discounts for payment in full to reduce cost.

- Based on prior credit approval, in-office financing terms of 3 months (interest-free)

- Interest-Free Dental financing. We have several companies that can finance up to $50,000 for care and in some cases even more based on your credit history. Subject to approval

- MasterCard or Visa time payments.

- Budgeting for your care over two years to make it more affordable.

- We also offer a "cruise plan." You pre-pay every two weeks until you build up a balance to start.

- Home equity loans; we can recommend several mortgage brokers to set this up.

- Loans from 401K/Pension plans (you pay yourself the interest); we can help start this process with your employer.

- Loans from life insurance/annuity policies; our accountant's office can help with this.

- Settling a Universal Life Policy that you or a family member no longer needs.

- Medical Savings account through an employer's cafeteria plan

- Gifts or Loans from friends or family members.

- Dental Insurance usually pays a maximum yearly benefit of $1,000-2,000 for your care.

- EXTERNAL Lines of Interest-Free Dental Credit are available *subject to approval*

- Medical Insurance rarely covers anything related to the mouth (I have only seen this one time!)

- In the highly unlikely event that your company administers its plan (self-insured employers), your company administrator might allow implant care; your company would know the specifics.

Dentistry is tax deductible for most patients. *Even if you finance your care, you can deduct the full amount in the year that you start treatment.* In fact, Uncle Sam's tax laws are in your favor to do your dental work as it is a legitimate medical deduction. Your tax adviser can help with this.

Obviously, costs vary considerably depending on your needs and desires. If you read all the letters we get from patients you will find that some people chose implants, rather than a cruise as an anniversary present to each other.

So yes, you will need to look at implants as an investment, because it is a significant decision. Implants truly are investments. A cruise or other trip ends after just a few days. Alternatively, you can purchase more "stuff" for the house, however, is that **as important as the very best appearance possible and the best possible health?**

A healthy mouth or magnificent dazzling smile pays dividends in many ways **for your entire life.** Dental Implants are admittedly not the least expensive option. If your primary concern is the cheapest price, then dental implants are not for you.

If, on the other hand, a reasonable investment and a fair price are important to you, but far more important is the best **possible outcome, the least pain and discomfort, the most gentle care and highest degree of expertise and professionalism,** then implants are for you. Incidentally, a variety of payments plans are available. Of course, all major credit cards are accepted so that you can get your airline miles or reward points. Some patients report getting five days' vacation at a top resort with the reward points on their credit card. We also offer 12-month interest-free plans. Expert assistance in obtaining reimbursements from your insurance provided free of charge.

Q: I want to know if I am a candidate, but I do not want to go to an office that is pushy or tries to sell me. What can I do?

A: Great Question. First, here's what I'd like to offer you:

A FREE Dental Implant and Healthy Smile Consultation!

When you contact us, we will invite you in for a 30-minute appointment, get some x-rays, look at your teeth and gums, and most importantly find out what **YOU WANT**. That is it.

If, at the end of the consultation, you do not feel like we can help you. That is fine. There is **NO PRESSURE** from us at all.

Why Wait?

The BEST DAY IS TODAY!

We are simply here to help you!

REGISTER

To receive more information, videos and downloads that will help you with Dental Implant Surgery visit:

www.DentalImplantsUtah.com
or
www.TrueDentistry.com

You can also schedule a speaking engagement or consulting session with Dr. Scott Hamblin.

ABOUT THE AUTHOR

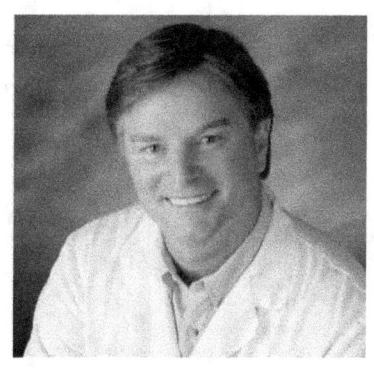

Scott Hamblin, D.D.S. is embracing the dramatic evolutions happening in dental care and treatment, and bringing them to his patients. His goal is to deliver the latest and best practices in ways that are consistent, comfortable and effective for his patients. He has been selected by Consumers Research Council of America as one of America's Top Dentists.

Dr. Hamblin was the team dentist for the Oakland A's professional baseball team for ten years. Dr. Hamblin has over 25 years experience as a practicing dentist in California, Utah, Nevada and Oregon giving him keen insights into what patients are seeking and how leading edge dentistry can fulfill those expectations. As an expert in implants, Dr. Hamblin teaches his techniques nationwide to other dentists. Dr. Hamblin is a graduate of Brigham Young University and Baylor College of Dentistry. His vast experience in aesthetics, implants, and sedation dentistry allows him to use the least invasive techniques and highest quality materials available. Dr. Hamblin is a member of *The International Congress of Oral Implantologists, The American Academy of Implant Dentistry and The American Dental Association.* He is *Invisalign Certified* and chosen as the *Salt Lake "Extreme Makeover" Dentist.* His unique cosmetic and implant dentistry has been featured on FOX News and ABC.

In his spare time Dr. Hamblin enjoys the outdoors: fly fishing, hiking, tennis, horseback riding, and biking. He also loves traveling with his wife, Linda. He is the father of 6 children and four grandchildren (many more to come!).

Follow Dr Hamblin:

Facebook: www.facebook.com/DentalImplantsUtah

Twitter: @mysldentist

Linkedin: www.linkedin.com/in/scott-hamblin-b697b661

YouTube: www.youtube.com/user/mysaltlakedentist

The End

www.ingramcontent.com/pod-product-compliance
Lightning Source LLC
Chambersburg PA
CBHW070142290526
45789CB00002B/594